Achieving an
AIDS Transition

Achieving an AIDS Transition

"Mead Over proposes a canny model for marshaling and coordinating donor contributions to AIDS prevention and treatment in developing countries. *Achieving an AIDS Transition* includes prudent and detailed plans that promise to bring us all closer to a transition long overdue."

PAUL FARMER, *Kolokotrones University Professor of Global Health and Social Medicine, Harvard University, and co-founder of Partners in Health*

"Living with AIDS is clearly better than dying with AIDS. But the best outcome is to return to an AIDS-free world. *Achieving an AIDS Transition* provides the essential foundation for understanding the transition."

PAUL COLLIER, *director of the Centre for the Study of African Economies, University of Oxford, and author of* The Bottom Billion

"There is an urgent need to take a long-term view on AIDS. *Achieving an AIDS Transition* is thought-provoking and provides an important contribution to this vital debate."

PETER PIOT, *director of the London School of Hygiene & Tropical Medicine and former executive director of UNAIDS*

"By examining the worldwide AIDS epidemic through the lens of economics, this book shows how donors and governments can look forward to the day when the burdens of AIDS and its treatment costs will be greatly reduced and increasingly affordable by national governments. I recommend this book to all who are looking for hard-headed analysis and a possible solution to the long-term sustainability of AIDS funding in severely affected countries."

PROFESSOR SIR RICHARD FEACHEM, *founding executive director of the Global Fund to Fight AIDS, Tuberculosis and Malaria, and executive director of Global Health Sciences, University of California–San Francisco*

"I highly recommend this book to those particularly concerned with a shared responsibility of tackling the AIDS epidemic in Africa. As sufficient donor funds are going to be increasingly harder to come by in these challenging global financial times, this book seeks a fresh set of ideas on how realignment of incentives between donors and our African governments and citizens can move us closer to self-sufficiency."

DAVID SERWADDA, *former dean of the Makerere School of Public Health, Uganda*

"At last, an innovative approach to stemming the flow of new HIV infections. Mead Over brings to our attention the importance of the AIDS transition and offers a hard-hitting, incentive-driven approach to HIV prevention."

MICHAEL MERSON, *director of the Duke Global Health Institute and former director of the WHO Global Program on AIDS*

"Mead Over is constructively provocative and someone whose thoughts deserve wide distribution and discussion."

JIMMY KOLKER, *chief of HIV/AIDS, UNICEF, and former deputy global AIDS coordinator, PEPFAR*

"Mead Over has proposed several ways that incentives can be used, at the national, local and individual levels, to improve the effectiveness of HIV prevention. His ideas are an important part of the global discussion as we search for innovative ways to sustain AIDS financing and slow the growth of the AIDS burden."

DAVID WILSON, *global AIDS program director, World Bank*

"*Achieving an AIDS Transition* gives hope to millions. This book is required reading for policymakers, researchers, students, and anyone interested in learning how the transition to a world free of AIDS can happen."

GERMANO MWABU, *professor of economics, University of Nairobi*

"Mead Over is one of the clearest thinkers in global health. He is also one of the few who has maintained an objective long-term view of the AIDS epidemic and, in stark contrast to many in the field, not shied away from articulating the consequences of inappropriate action."

RIFAT ATUN, *professor of international health management, Imperial College London, and director of the Strategy, Performance, and Evaluation Cluster, Global Fund to Fight AIDS, Tuberculosis and Malaria*

Achieving an AIDS Transition

Preventing Infections to Sustain Treatment

Mead Over

CENTER FOR GLOBAL DEVELOPMENT
Washington, D.C.

Achieving an AIDS Transition: Preventing Infections to Sustain Treatment
may be ordered from:
BROOKINGS INSTITUTION PRESS
c/o HFS, P.O. Box 50370, Baltimore, MD 21211-4370
Tel.: 800/537-5487; 410/516-6956; Fax: 410/516-6998; Internet: www.brookings.edu

CGD is grateful for contributions from The Bill & Melinda Gates Foundation
in support of this work.

Library of Congress Cataloging-in-Publication data
Over, A. Mead.
   Achieving an AIDS transition : preventing infections to sustain treatment /
Mead Over.
      p.;   cm.
   Includes bibliographical references and index.
   ISBN 978-1-933286-38-9 (pbk. : alk. paper)—ISBN 978-1-933286-62-4 (e-book)
1. AIDS (Disease)—Prevention.   I. Title.
   [DNLM: 1. HIV Infections—prevention & control.   2. Acquired
Immunodeficiency Syndrome—prevention & control.   WC 503.6]
   RC607.A26O93 2011
   616.97'92—dc22   2011000619

9 8 7 6 5 4 3 2 1

Printed on acid-free paper

Typeset in Sabon and Myriad

Composition by R. Lynn Rivenbark
Macon, Georgia

Printed by R. R. Donnelley
Harrisonburg, Virginia

Cover photo: AIDS orphans in the Biwi/Mchesi area of Lilongwe, Malawi. Some rights
reserved by Flickr user khym54 under the Creative Commons Attribution 2.0 license.

Contents

Appendixes

Preface

Can an economist's perspective help to justify greater expenditure on controlling the AIDS epidemic? When the late Dr. Jonathan Mann, the first head of the Global Program on AIDS, approached me at the World Bank in 1987 with that question, I had only an inkling of how big a problem AIDS would become for the developing world in general and for Africa in particular. Nor could I imagine that donors would spend so many billions of dollars on AIDS—only to see the need for money grow even faster.

At a 2005 summit conference in Gleneagles, Scotland, the G-8 leaders, perhaps encouraged by the billions of dollars newly authorized by the United States to fund the President's Emergency Plan for AIDS Relief (PEPFAR), pledged to assure universal access to AIDS treatment by 2010. But after years of double-digit increases reaching a high of $7.7 billion dollars in 2008, donor disbursements for AIDS stabilized in 2009 at $7.6 billion and are unlikely to increase in the next few years. This scaling back in donor ambitions is happening despite the continued increase of the number of people living with HIV/AIDS, which in 2010 surpassed 33 million.

One possible future is that donors will turn away from AIDS, reducing their budget allocations and expenditures year-by-year. Under this scenario, the grand humanitarian commitments to vanquish AIDS in poor countries will be gradually and quietly abandoned—just as the goal of malaria eradication was abandoned a few decades ago.

That would be a tragedy. Failure in the struggle against AIDS at this point would spread despair among the people suffering from HIV infection and their families. A failure of AIDS assistance would also have implications for foreign assistance more generally. The taxpayers in rich countries would be justified in asking why the foreign policy elite have failed to accomplish their stated goal of universal access to AIDS treatment. Was it because meeting the needs of poor people in poor countries is a reckless and foolish ambition—that we will always have poverty and disease? Will that reinforce the suspicion that foreign aid cannot be counted on for results— with potentially tragic consequences for the future of millions who could be helped by aid-financed programs?

In this book, Mead Over, senior fellow at the Center for Global Development since 2006, former Peace Corps volunteer, economics professor at Williams College and Boston University, World Bank economist, and one of world's leading economic specialists on the AIDS epidemic, presents a vision for a "win" on AIDS policy—a hopeful alternative to the abandonment that otherwise might lie ahead. His controversial but realistic proposal is that AIDS prevention be the horse that pulls the cart, generating an "AIDS transition" analogous to the demographic transition donors successfully supported three decades ago in the developing world. He lays out, among other approaches to prevention, the logic and the implication of using some portion of AIDS funding to pay governments directly for measured reductions in the incidence of new HIV infections.

Getting to the AIDS transition, the milestone after which the number of people living with HIV/AIDS begins to decline, does not itself constitute a "win" against this devastating epidemic. But it's a stepping-stone to that objective, which if explicitly sought, will help donors and governments justify continued expenditure in the short run and to plan reasonably and confidently for the end of both the depredation and the burden of this scourge.

NANCY BIRDSALL
President
Center for Global Development

Acknowledgments

This book is the distillation of twenty-five years of work on the economics of AIDS, so my debts of gratitude extend deep into the past and far across the world.

First, I thank Jonathan Mann, whose 1987 request to the World Bank for technical assistance in estimating the economic impact of AIDS led him to invite me to spend three years working with the Global Programme on AIDS, the ancestor of UNAIDS, on the economic impact of the AIDS epidemic. I thank Nancy Birdsall, the president of the Center for Global Development and the author of the preface to this book, who was then the chief of the health economics research unit at the World Bank, for designating me then to work on the topic and for supporting my work on this book here at the CGD since my arrival.

Thanks to my World Bank supervisors, Ann Hamilton, Anthony Measham, Dean Jamison, Emmanuel Jimenez, Paul Collier, David Wheeler, Zmarak Shalizi, and Ritva Reinikka, who supported my AIDS economics work at the World Bank. There, under the insightful supervision of Lyn Squire, I had the pleasure of applying the economics lens to AIDS with my good friend and colleague Martha Ainsworth as we produced *Confronting AIDS: Public Priorities in a Global Epidemic*. I appreciate the continuing collaboration and support over the years from current and former World Bank colleagues Nicholas Prescott, Jacques van der Gaag, Hans Binswanger, Lawrence MacDonald, Richard Skolnik, Miriam Schneidman,

Timothy Johnston, Damien de Walque, Susan Stout, David Wilson, Robert Oelrichs, Jody Kusek, William McGreevey, and Phil Musgrove.

Tanzanian research collaborators Phare Mujinja, Godlike Koda, George Lwihula, and Innocent Semali and project manager Tom Wayman taught me about how households cope with AIDS. Thanks to Peter Piot, King Holmes, James Chin, Nancy Padian, Sevgi Aral, Geoffrey Garnett, Timothy Hallett, and Julian Gold for introducing me to the complexities of HIV prevention, HIV epidemiological modeling, and antiretroviral therapy.

I appreciate the opportunity offered me by Jacky Mathonnet and Martine Audibert to try out my ideas and models on their students in their master's program in health economics at the University of the Auvergne. And thanks to Stefano Bertozzi, Hnin Hnin Pyne, Julia Dayton, Indrani Gupta, Kathleen Beegle, Daniel Dorsainvil, Mattias Lundberg, Emiko Masaki, Martina Tonizzo, Owen McCarthy, and Tejaswi Velayudhan, who over the years have helped me struggle not only with the conceptual puzzles arising out of the substance of the work, but also with Stata, data, and manuscripts.

I've benefited greatly from the views of CGD's global health experts— Ruth Levine, Rachel Nugent, Nandini Oomman, William Savedoff, and Amanda Glassman—as well as experts on other development topics. I appreciate the critical perspectives on my work offered by Angus Deaton, Anne Case, Charles Holmes, John Blandford, Greg Gonsalves, David Barr, and Jimmy Kolker, though I have not always been convinced by their arguments. Additional thanks go to John Osterman and Laura Wallace, who supported the production of this book in its last stages. I am grateful to the Bill & Melinda Gates Foundation for its financial support of this work.

And special thanks to my wife, Elizabeth King, and my daughters, Alexandra and Veronica, who have tolerated my business trips and listened with appropriate skepticism to my latest theories for so many years on the same topic. I hope that my daughters will see AIDS transitions become commonplace in country after country around the world, so that the scourge of this disease finally disappears from the planet.

Achieving an
AIDS Transition

CHAPTER 1

The Global AIDS Transition:
A Feasible Objective for AIDS Policy

About 1.8 million people died from AIDS-related illnesses in 2009; 1.6 million were adults in the prime of life.[1] Meanwhile, about 2.6 million people were newly infected with HIV, thus increasing the total number of people living with HIV/AIDS by more than 750,000.[2] With 33.3 million people living with HIV/AIDS at the end of 2009, the burden of this epidemic continues to grow with every passing year.

In this book, I propose a new paradigm for combating the HIV/AIDS epidemic and a new objective around which international donors and recipient governments can coordinate their efforts. I call this objective the "AIDS transition." In this chapter, I define the AIDS transition and show how adopting it as an objective can eventually eliminate the burden of the HIV/AIDS epidemic on the world. In the second chapter, I address the challenge of reducing new HIV infections sufficiently to bring about an AIDS transition. Recognizing the accumulating burden of supporting AIDS patients in low-income countries, I consider in the third chapter how donors and governments can sustain the success of AIDS treatment at a pace that will prevent a resurgence of AIDS deaths.

What exactly is an "AIDS transition"? It is a dynamic process that preserves recently achieved AIDS mortality reductions while lowering the number of new infections even further so that the total number of people living with HIV/AIDS diminishes. Once the total number of people living with HIV/AIDS begins to decline in a country, access to universal treatment

1

will get closer to becoming a reality every passing year—instead of receding as it has recently. And a future without AIDS will become a reasonable goal instead of the fantasy it seems today.

Here I first define the AIDS transition in more detail, comparing it to the demographic transition that played a prominent role in development during the twentieth century. I find harbingers of an AIDS transition in the recent epidemiological trends reported by the World Health Organization (WHO) and UNAIDS, the Joint United Nations Program on HIV/AIDS. I provide calculations of when and how the transition might occur, and I conclude by discussing policy opportunities that emerge from the AIDS transition perspective.

Defining an "AIDS Transition"

As the third decade of the AIDS epidemic marches on, remarkable successes at extending treatment to millions and a few signs of progress in prevention are overshadowed by a single stark statistic: for every person placed on AIDS treatment in 2009, about two new HIV cases arose.[3] Thus, the epidemic continues to spread faster than it can be prevented or treated through the combined efforts of all donors.

In view of the extraordinary rate at which AIDS patients in low- and middle-income countries have enrolled in antiretroviral therapy (ART) programs since 2003—from less than 100,000 in 2003 to more 6 million at the end of 2010—an optimist might see the continued excess of new infections over new enrollments as a temporary phenomenon. But this view ignores not only the swelling human cost of the increasing numbers of people dependent on a daily drug for survival, but also the fiscal implications, which are even less sustainable given the worsened financial environment that has resulted from the global economic crisis. For the United States, which provides about half of all donor support to AIDS treatment through its President's Emergency Plan for AIDS Relief (PEPFAR), the cost of treating all who need it in the fifteen original target countries would absorb half of U.S. foreign assistance funds by the year 2016 (Over 2009b). Since limited foreign assistance resources in the United States and other countries also will be needed for other foreign policy objectives, now is the time to reframe the challenge presented by the global AIDS epidemic.

This chapter proposes a new paradigm for combating AIDS, one focused on sustaining an AIDS transition, which will occur in two phases. The first milestone is when the number of new HIV/AIDS infections in a country's population falls below the number of deaths from AIDS, so that the total number of people living with HIV/AIDS begins to fall. But if new infections are only slightly fewer than deaths, the total number of people with AIDS will fall very slowly. Backsliding on prevention or improved treatment technology could reverse the situation a year later. As a result, the AIDS transition truly will be consolidated only after the number of new infections is kept below continually suppressed AIDS deaths for about a decade. Only then will the number of people living with HIV/AIDS decline enough so that the disease takes its place among treatable chronic diseases such as diabetes, cancer, and heart disease.

The development and deployment of an effective vaccine to prevent new infections would shorten dramatically the road to an AIDS transition. But three decades of experience have shown that HIV poses an extraordinarily difficult challenge to the immune system and to those who would prepare a vaccine to fend off the virus. Time and again, the goal of an effective vaccine has appeared within reach, only to vanish like a mirage as we have approached. That said, researchers must continue to pursue this elusive goal, and if we are lucky, their findings will yield biological insights that also will benefit other diseases.

For the foreseeable future, however, HIV prevention will depend on solving the social problem arising from the simple fact that for many people, the individual threat of developing AIDS—because it is uncertain and would only occur years later—seems insufficient to counterbalance the immediate rewards from unprotected sexual intercourse and needle-sharing intravenous drug use, which drive the epidemic (see box 1-1). These risks, taken by individuals, impose massive costs on the entire society in the form of a fiscal burden, medical dependency, and an increased threat of future infection to every sexually maturing young adult—indeed, to children everywhere. We all need to work together to ensure an AIDS transition through available interventions, without depending on a vaccine discovery that may never occur.[4]

Figure 1-1 helps us visualize the history of AIDS with a stylized version of the AIDS epidemic in a typical highly affected country. The solid lines in both panels represent the past, and the dashed lines represent the hoped-for future. When the epidemic began, the number of new infections was greater than the number of deaths of AIDS patients (see panel a), reflecting the fact that many years usually pass before HIV-infected individuals become sick and die. This led to a rapidly rising number of people with HIV/AIDS (panel b). As the epidemic matured, the annual number of

BOX 1-1. A Snapshot of AIDS Treatment

Because HIV is a retrovirus, it can only be treated with antiretroviral therapy (ART). To combat drug resistance, this medication is typically dispensed as a mixture of three different drugs, called combination or triple-drug therapy. The price of first-line ART has fallen dramatically over the years and is now available as a low-cost generic drug—heavily subsidized in the developing world by foreign donors. The tricky part of the treatment is that the drugs must be taken every day, and sometimes several times a day, for the rest of the patient's life. If the patient fails to adhere closely to the prescribed timing and dosages, a drug-resistant strain of HIV will develop. At that point, the patient will either die within months or shift to a new and typically much more expensive drug or combination of drugs known as second-line treatment. This treatment is not available in a generic form or funded by donors.

At what point are HIV-infected patients supposed to begin taking ART? In contrast to most other infectious diseases, HIV/AIDS takes years to make a person sick. The time from infection to illness is typically about eight years but can vary from five to twelve years or more. Once a patient begins first-line therapy, he or she can postpone mortality by four to ten years. If first-line therapy fails, second-line treatment can postpone mortality for another two to ten years.

A key measure of the progression of HIV is the number of CD4 cells per microliter of the patient's blood, a count that declines from nearly 1,000 for uninfected people to zero as the person's immune system is destroyed by HIV. Until recently, the World Health Organization recommended that patients begin treatment for AIDS once their cell count reaches 200 cells per microliter, or about eight years after becoming infected. In 2009, however, the organization revised its guidelines, recommending that treatment begin a year or more earlier, when the CD4 count has dropped to 350 cells per microliter of blood (WHO 2009).

These guidelines will be very expensive to adopt. Although the number receiving subsidized AIDS treatment in low- and middle-income countries, mostly in sub-Saharan Africa, has risen from a few thousand people in 2003 to about 6 million in 2010, about 57 percent of those in need are going untreated. At the 350 threshold, current coverage would drop to a dismal 30–40 percent, a far cry from the global community's goal of universal coverage.

FIGURE 1-1. Achieving an AIDS Transition: A Milestone on the Road to a World without AIDS

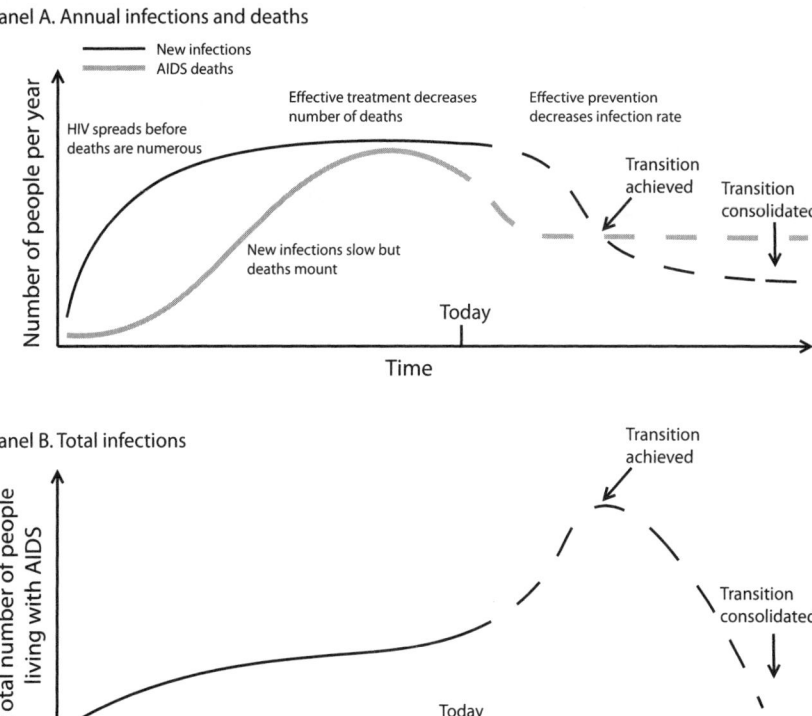

Panel A. Annual infections and deaths

Panel B. Total infections

Source: Author's construction.

new infections (the incidence of HIV) did not change very much, but the annual number of deaths eventually rose almost as high, slowing the rate of growth of the population living with AIDS (the prevalence of HIV/AIDS).[5]

Then, beginning in 2000, an increasing proportion of AIDS patients started ART, which began to slow the number of deaths. At the same time, the annual number of new infections declined slowly because prevention efforts were insufficient and ineffective. The result has been a dramatic rise in the number of people living with HIV/AIDS. If we do not change our approach, the gap between these two flows—AIDS patients dying and new individuals becoming infected—will continue to widen, producing a "population explosion" of AIDS patients.

What can be done? The goal should be twofold: (1) to suppress the annual number of deaths by continued access to effective treatment; and (2) to reduce the annual number of new infections over the next few years by effective HIV prevention. As figure 1-1 shows, when a country succeeds in pushing new infections down below the number of annual deaths, it will succeed in achieving the first AIDS transition milestone. And after many years of further efforts to sustain access to quality treatment and suppress new infections, the total number of people with HIV/AIDS will decline to levels not seen since the beginning of the epidemic. At that point, the country will have consolidated its AIDS transition, and universal access to AIDS treatment will be financially feasible for even the poorest countries.

But neither the decades-old origin of the AIDS epidemic nor the decades-in-the-future eventual consolidation of the AIDS transition are of as much interest to us today as the immediate future. Figure 1-2 focuses on the time-slice of figure 1-1 starting a few years ago, when effective AIDS treatment began to reduce annual deaths, and then extends to only a few years from now, when we might reach the attainable milestone of the AIDS transition. The figure emphasizes that if the AIDS transition succeeds, the current surge of people living with HIV/AIDS will be temporary, slowing when annual numbers of new infections decline. In the year when new infections first fall below the annual number of deaths, the total number of people living with HIV/AIDS will have peaked, and the focus will turn toward consolidating the transition.

A Dynamic Transition

The AIDS transition has commonalities with another transition in the history of public health: the demographic transition, when a largely rural agrarian society with high fertility and mortality rates shifted to a predominantly urban industrial society with low fertility and mortality rates (Thompson 1929; Coale 1973; Hammer and others 2008).[6] Both transitions are dynamic processes with great momentum; they begin with a threatening "population explosion" because of declining mortality; and stopping them requires slowing the trend that fuels that explosion (reducing births in the case of population and infections in the case of AIDS). Neither is amenable to a quick fix—averting the explosions by allowing mortality to rise would have tragic human consequences and generate politically unacceptable reputational risks for donors and perhaps governments (Over 2009b).

In the AIDS transition, dynamism is evident at many levels. For the population, risky behaviors that spread HIV ebb and flow in response not only

FIGURE 1-2. The Number of Patients on Antiretroviral Therapy (ART) Will Grow before a Transition Takes Hold

Panel A. Annual infections and deaths

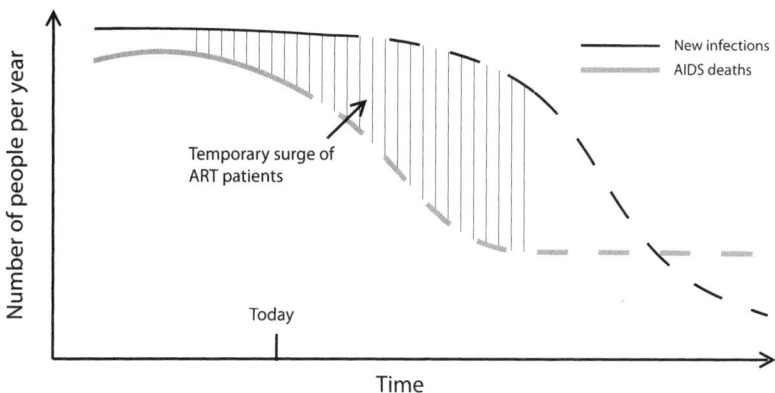

Panel B. Total infections

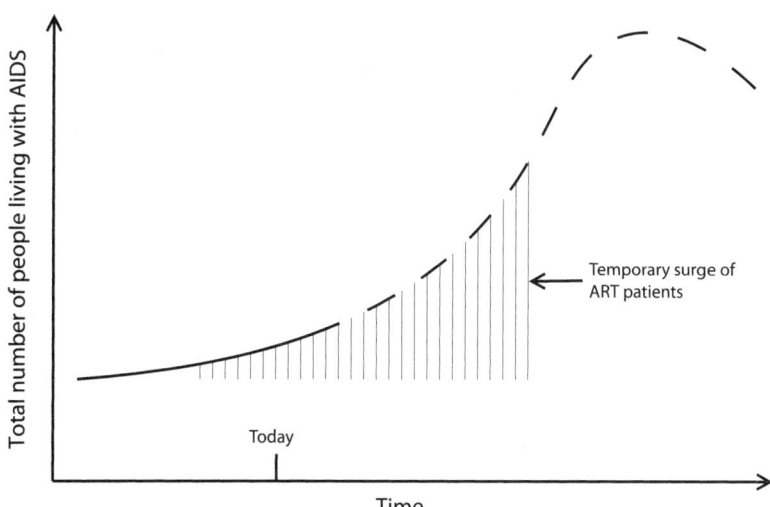

Source: Over 2004.

to population dynamics and economic growth patterns, but also to the changing perception of the riskiness of those behaviors. In turn, HIV transmission ebbs and flows in response to behavioral cycles. Within each patient, the billions of replicating virus particles surge, then ebb, then surge again as the virus fights a years-long war of attrition with the host's immune system.[7] Even society's responses—including fear; denial; recognition; and policies to prevent, treat, and mitigate the disease's impact—ebb and flow in response to changing political personalities, fluctuating donor fashions, new cohorts of youth coming of age, and the boom and bust of economic cycles.

That said, the AIDS transition and the demographic transition also have many differences. In the demographic transition, despite concerns about the pressure that a high birth rate puts on our limited resources, each individual baby is a cause for celebration. Furthermore, a population boom causes a bulge in the age distribution of many countries, which in turn contributes a "demographic gift" in the form of increased savings and faster economic growth when that wave of people enters the labor force (Bloom and Williamson 1998).

In contrast, a new case of HIV infection leads to pain, suffering, premature death, and serious economic consequences. Each additional AIDS patient treated with subsidized ART, no matter how successfully, will draw down national saving by the amount of his or her domestically financed treatment subsidy. Even patients who pay for their own care are diverting private resources away from consumption and investment, as well as scarce medical resources away from other competing health needs.

Moreover, in the demographic transition, as adults learn that their children are less likely to die in childhood, they desire fewer children. A decline in desired family size, if supported with family planning information and supplies, leads to a decline in birth rates.

But in the AIDS transition, the impact on new infections of AIDS treatment access and the consequently smaller number of deaths is more complicated and less clearly desirable. As table 1-1 shows, treatment has a mix of behavioral and biological effects. Just as awareness of lower childhood mortality reduces peoples' fear that their children will die and thus gives them the confidence to plan fewer children, awareness of lower AIDS mortality has reduced peoples' fear of knowing their HIV infection status and thus encouraged them to seek testing and treatment at an earlier stage of the disease. Effective treatment also reduces new infections by lowering the number of virus particles in bodily fluids, thereby reducing the rate of transmission associated with potential exposures.[8]

Unfortunately, pernicious effects in both the biological and the behavioral dimensions offset the desirable effects of treatment on the number of new infections. In the biological dimension, ART can select resistant strains of HIV, which can replicate in, and be spread by, ART patients (Friedland and Williams 1999; Bangsberg and others 2003). And because treatment

TABLE 1-1. AIDS Treatment Affects HIV Transmission, but Not Always in a Good Way

	Effects that might slow transmission	*Effects that might speed transmission*
Biological	Reduces viral load in the HIV-infected person, which reduces the infectivity of each sexual contact	Lengthens duration of infectivity, which increases number of contacts
		Selects for resistant strains of HIV, which can be transmitted despite the presence of antiretroviral drugs
Behavioral	Motivates HIV testing, but testing has an ambiguous impact on transmission	Reduces perceived danger of unsafe behavior, potentially leading to the "disinhibition" of risk behavior that had previously been inhibited by fear of AIDS.
	Promotes solidarity and reduces the stigma associated with HIV/AIDS, which might facilitate prevention campaigns in some settings	

Source: Over and others 2004.

lengthens patients' lives, it obviously lengthens the time during which these patients can infect others.

On the behavioral side, the increased HIV testing resulting from wider treatment access has been a mixed blessing for HIV prevention. People who have learned that they are HIV positive subsequently report reducing their risky sexual contacts. However, since they are aware that society expects this of them, their self-reported behavior might belie a less altruistic change in behavior in the other direction. On the other hand, people who test negative actually report an increase in risky behavior, especially if they have tested negative several times (Sherr and others 2007).[9]

Furthermore, the very effectiveness and accessibility of AIDS treatment naturally reduce peoples' fear of the disease. Given that risky sex and intravenous drug use are inherently gratifying, people are rational to increase those behaviors in response to the perception that the consequences are less dangerous. Such perverse effects in association with AIDS treatment have occurred in various settings around the world, including Nairobi, Kenya, and several American and European cities (Miller and others 2000; Katz and others 2002). To quote UNAIDS, "HIV incidence appears to be either stable or on the rise in numerous countries where antiretroviral therapy has long been widely available" (WHO, UNAIDS, and UNICEF 2009, p. 18).

Another way the two transitions differ is in whether economic development helps or hinders. Although the demographic transition is not yet complete in all parts of the world, population death rates have generally remained low, and birth rates have continued to decline. As countries urbanize, educate the female population, and improve the availability of family planning information and supplies, people seem to want to reduce their fertility rates to approximately replacement level. The momentum of development is clearly reinforcing government policy in the direction of a successful demographic transition.

In contrast, countries severely affected by AIDS have no perceptible development-related momentum for the AIDS transition. Although significantly suppressed by vigorous government- and donor-supported AIDS treatment programs in many low- and middle-income countries, AIDS mortality would bounce back up again within months if these subsidized programs were removed. And in low-income countries, the number of HIV infections shows no sign of declining "naturally" in response to expanded access to AIDS treatment (WHO, UNAIDS, and UNICEF 2009).

Many Ways to Fail

What are the chances of success with the AIDS transition? Sadly, they are uncertain at best. Granted, the spread of AIDS treatment has launched the first stage of AIDS transition in many countries, but the transition can fail just as ignobly as did the last century's plan to eradicate malaria. In 1955 the WHO announced a worldwide Global Malaria Eradication Program, only to admit defeat in 1969 (Tanner and de Savigny 2008). Some forty years later, the Global Roll Back Malaria Program is gaining momentum—but notably without the word "eradication" in its title.

So what form might failure take? Three possible scenarios stand out in which the number of people living with HIV/AIDS would continue to grow unimpeded rather than eventually decrease, as illustrated in figure 1-1. One involves treatment failure, and all involve prevention failure. They all lead to ever-faster accumulations of the population undergoing treatment with ART until, by the arithmetic of compound interest, keeping them alive requires an ever-growing portion of the total resources of the health sector and then of society as a whole.

In the first scenario, donors and governments not only fail to reduce the number of newly infected individuals, but also fail to sustain the quality and the number of people recruited as new ART patients, which, in turn, influences the number of AIDS deaths. As a result, the current surge in the number living with HIV/AIDS would initially slow but then continue to grow. While the growth rate in the total number of people with HIV/AIDS would be slowest with this type of transition failure, the resurgence in AIDS mortality would resemble the resurgence of malaria deaths throughout sub-Saharan Africa and Asia after the Global Malaria Eradication effort was terminated in 1969 (Packard 1997). The failure would be depressing—even humiliating—and would discredit all involved with the effort to widen access to AIDS treatment.

In the second possible scenario, donors and governments sustain the quality and the number of people recruited as new ART patients, but they fail to slow the incidence of new infections. In this case, the continued "success" of treatment would lead inevitably to immense fatigue as donors and governments became overwhelmed with the burden of maintaining constantly growing numbers of people on treatment.

In the third scenario, donors and governments again sustain the quality and the number of people recruited as new ART patients but fail so miserably on the prevention front that the incidence of new infections actually rises. Among the three types of AIDS transition failure, this one would lead to the most explosive growth of people living with HIV/AIDS. It would occur if the net impact of AIDS treatment is to stimulate rather than depress HIV transmission.

Which of these scenarios is most likely to occur? Given the current slowdown in the availability of funding for AIDS treatment and the lack of progress toward effective HIV prevention, the most likely transition failure is the first scenario. If AIDS deaths eventually rise—which would reflect either a cessation of patient recruitment or a lowering of treatment standards—we can expect AIDS treatment providers, beneficiaries, and advocates to loudly blame one another and the rest of the foreign assistance community for this reversal. In the minds of tax-paying constituents in donor countries, the ensuing acrimony is likely to tarnish the entire AIDS-assistance enterprise, reducing AIDS donors' ability to fund AIDS treatment or prevention. Indeed, public disappointment with the reversal of the much-celebrated recent mortality reductions might engender the feeling that *any* kind of foreign assistance is ultimately hopeless, thus leading to a loss of public support for foreign assistance funding in general. For these reasons, the feasible objective of the AIDS transition benefits not only the AIDS community, but all those with an interest in the foreign assistance enterprise.

A New Policy Tool

A new paradigm alone is no magic bullet for the AIDS epidemic. The litmus test of the paradigm will be whether it enables all policymakers—from national leaders to the municipal authorities, from heads of donor agencies to those who negotiate and implement project agreements—to integrate the twin goals of reducing mortality through treatment and preventing new infections. Any program that accomplishes one goal but not the other must be called to account. Only programs that work on both—and can show results on both—should be eligible for funding.

Harbingers of an AIDS Transition

How far along is the global community on the AIDS transition? The answer is that the world as a whole—and sub-Saharan Africa in particular—is only in the initial stages.

As figure 1-3 shows, Africa is experiencing the most marked mortality reduction of any region in the world, characteristic of the beginning of an AIDS transition. Annual deaths declined from 1.6 million in 2005 to 1.4 million in 2008, a drop of 4.5 percent per year. This continent-wide average hides even greater declines in some countries. Between 2002 and 2006, AIDS mortality in Kenya fell by 29 percent, or at an annual rate of 7 percent per year (National AIDS Control Council 2007).

The mortality trend for Asia also looks hopeful, as India, the country with the most AIDS cases, rolls out AIDS treatment to an increasingly large percentage of those who need it. However, the annual number of AIDS deaths has not yet begun to decline in Latin America and continues to rise in Eastern Europe and Central Asia. Although Brazil, Argentina, Poland, and a few other countries in these regions have taken great strides toward mortality reduction, the regions in aggregate have not yet achieved the mortality reductions that are the harbinger of the first stage of an AIDS transition.

On the prevention side—the other half of the transition story—sub-Saharan Africa and Asia accounted for 84 percent of the roughly 2.7 million new infections in 2008. Moreover, as table 1-2 shows, new HIV infections continue to exceed the number of deaths from AIDS in about 86 percent of the 97 developing countries for which we have estimates.[10] In other words, these countries are only in the initial phase of an AIDS transition. The worry is whether and how quickly they will proceed to the next stage. Even such countries as Brazil, Mexico, and Senegal, which have some of the best HIV-prevention programs in the world, have not been able to lower the number of new infections below AIDS mortality. Other countries, including South Africa and Zambia, have achieved heroic expansion of ART access from 2007–2008 but have not shown evidence of better prevention.

The 15 percent of developing countries where AIDS deaths exceed new infections are worth noting (see table 1-3). Rwanda and Cambodia are in

FIGURE 1-3. Estimated Number of AIDS Deaths with and without Antiretroviral Therapy, 1996–2008 (thousands)

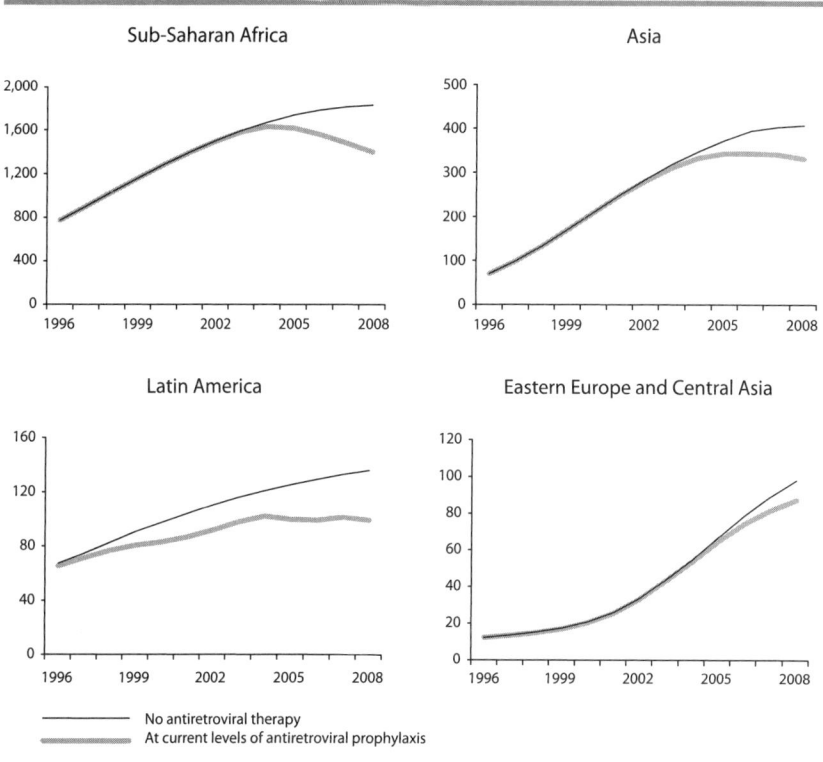

Source: WHO, UNAIDS, and UNICEF 2009.

the forefront of the AIDS transition. If they can sustain their 90 percent treatment coverage and hold incidence rates below lowered death rates, they may be the first countries to consolidate the transition. India, Uganda, Zimbabwe, and Burkina Faso also seem to be on the way to consolidating the AIDS transition, for two reasons: they have made impressive reductions in incidence from previously much higher levels, and they have not expanded AIDS treatment as much as some other countries. It is critical that the incidence reductions be sustained as they strive to expand treatment coverage. In Uganda, the most frequently cited example of successful prevention, worrisome evidence shows that the rate of risky behavior and HIV infection in antenatal clinics are rising (Opio and others 2008; Guwatudde and others 2009). In Côte d'Ivoire, Myanmar, and Burundi, AIDS treatment coverage is so low at under one-third that their AIDS

TABLE 1-2. Estimated New HIV Infections, AIDS Deaths, and Patients on Antiretroviral Therapy (ART) in Selected Countries where New Infections Exceed Deaths, 2007–08

Country	Estimated new HIV infections in 2007	Deaths in 2007	Percentage of new infections that exceed deaths	Patients on ART in 2008	Percent increase in ART 2007–08	Estimated percent of coverage in 2008
South Africa	432,857	350,000	23.7	701,000	52.4	39.3
Nigeria	231,428	170,000	36.1	239,000	20.7	29.5
Kenya	195,000	107,500	81.4	243,000	37.3	43.6
Zambia	103,500	56,000	84.8	226,000	49.7	59.9
Ethiopia	93,642	67,000	39.8	132,000	46.7	39.2
Thailand	39,071	30,000	30.2	180,000	17.6	69.5
Vietnam	36,614	24,000	52.6	27,100	59.4	34.0
Brazil	23,857	15,000	59.0	190,000	5.0	79.5
Angola	20,635	11,000	87.6	13,000	8.3	23.0
Colombia	14,828	9,800	51.3	23,100	10.0	39.1
Namibia	14,528	5,100	184.9	59,000	13.5	82.5
Swaziland	14,500	10,000	45.0	32,700	30.8	51.5
Botswana	14,200	11,000	29.1	117,000	25.8	95.0
Haiti	11,707	7,200	62.6	19,300	28.7	47.6

Sources: Deaths in 2007 and patients on ART are from UNAIDS 2008; WHO, UNAIDS, and UNICEF 2009. Estimates of incidence are computed by the author from The Joint United Nations Program on HIV/AIDS (UNAIDS) and World Health Organization time-series data on prevalence, deaths, and treatment rollout by country. Estimated coverage in 2008 is defined as the ratio of the number of 2008 ART patients to the sum of 2008 ART patients and need in 2007, according to UNAIDS's 2007 methodology. Selected countries have a ratio of estimated incidence to deaths greater than 1.2, a ratio of enrolled ART patients to the total number needing ART in 2007 greater than 0.25, and an estimated number of incident cases greater than 5,000.

deaths have not yet fallen below the rate of new infections. As they work to expand treatment coverage, they can prevent the surge in the total number of people living with HIV/AIDS by simultaneously improving prevention effectiveness. In this way, they can move more directly and immediately to consolidate an AIDS transition.

Uneasy Early Victories

Another way to track progress on the AIDS transition is to step back and look at the time paths of new HIV infections since 1980. At first glance, the news from Asia and sub-Saharan Africa seems promising given that the number of new infections appears to be slightly declining (see figure 1-4). For the period 2001–2008, when accuracy might be highest, UNAIDS estimates that the declines in the number of new infections have been at the annual rate of 1.9 percent in Asia and 2.7 percent per year in Africa. Perhaps if these trends are simply sustained, the number of new infections will eventually fall below the number of annual deaths, and the number of people living with HIV/AIDS will begin to decline.

TABLE 1-3. Estimated New HIV Infections, AIDS Deaths, and Patients on Antiretroviral Therapy (ART) in All Countries where Deaths Exceed New Infections, 2007–2008

Country	Estimated new HIV infections in 2007	Deaths in 2007	Percentage of new infections that exceed deaths[1]	Patients on ART in 2008	Percent increase in ART 2007–08	Estimated percent of coverage in 2008
India	196,733	213,677	−7.9	235,000	48.7	30.0
Uganda	64,357	77,000	−16.4	164,000	42.6	48.6
Zimbabwe	53,571	140,000	−61.7	148,000	51.0	30.6
Cote d'Ivoire	23,357	38,000	−38.5	52,000	0.0	29.7
Myanmar	14,000	25,000	−44.0	15,200	38.2	23.4
Burundi	7,428	11,000	−32.5	14,000	27.3	32.2
Burkina Faso	7,257	9,200	−21.1	21,100	24.1	45.8
Rwanda	6,985	7,800	−10.4	63,000	28.6	93.8
Honduras	1,700	1,900	−10.5	6,300	12.5	53.4
Cambodia	1,400	6,900	−79.7	32,000	18.5	92.8
Djibouti	814	1,100	−26.0	999	42.7	23.7
Belarus	385	1,100	−65.0	1,200	33.3	33.5
Gambia	370	401	−7.7	999	100.2	44.0

Sources: Columns with deaths and patients on ART are from UNAIDS 2008; WHO, UNAIDS, and UNICEF 2009. Estimates of incidence are computed by the author from The Joint United Nations Program on HIV/AIDS (UNAIDS) and World Health Organization time-series data on prevalence, deaths, and treatment rollout by country. Estimated coverage in 2008 is defined as the ratio of the number of 2008 ART patients to the sum of 2008 ART patients and need in 2007, according to UNAIDS's 2007 methodology.

1. Negative numbers in column three indicate that deaths exceed new infections.

For example, if Asia were to remain on its current trajectory, the number of people living with HIV/AIDS in Asia would begin declining in 2015. But given the continued dramatic expansion of ART in India, China, and Vietnam—and the likelihood that Thailand and Cambodia will sustain or even further expand treatment access—AIDS mortality is likely to fall even faster. By taking preemptive action on HIV prevention, the region can avoid an explosion in the number of people living with HIV/AIDS, moving more quickly to the consolidation stage, in which AIDS is a manageable, rarely infectious, chronic disease.

In sub-Saharan Africa, AIDS mortality has been falling by 4.5 percent a year, more than twice as fast as the decline in new infections, creating a population explosion of people living with HIV/AIDS. Moreover, evidence shows that the incidence decline has slowed and perhaps even stabilized. Determining what will happen next is difficult: debate continues over how much of the decline in incidence has been caused by changes in risk behavior as a result of government- and donor-funded prevention interventions—and how much would have occurred anyway owing to the natural evolutionary pattern of any infectious disease epidemic. For example, the massive

FIGURE 1-4. Annual Incidence of New HIV Infections by Region, 1990–2008 (thousands)

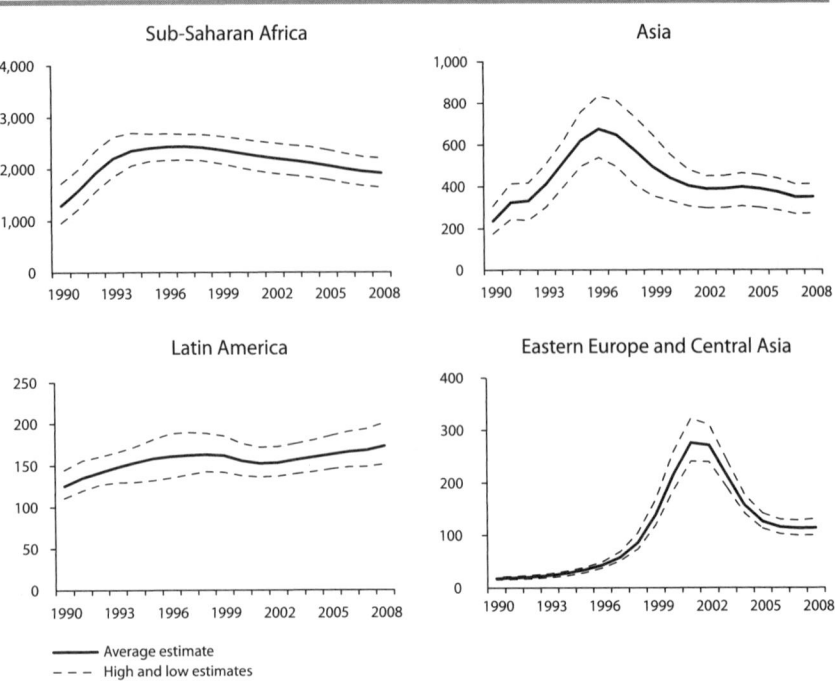

Source: WHO, UNAIDS, and UNICEF 2009.

expenditures of the PEPFAR program in Africa since 2003, while coinciding with the decline in mortality rate on that continent (figure 1-3), do not seem to have been associated with any traceable decline in new HIV infections (figure 1-4). While hardly strong evidence against the effectiveness of PEP-FAR prevention efforts, this observation suggests that recent declines in HIV incidence might be cyclical and subject to reversal.

A recent study by Imperial College London's Dr. Timothy Hallett and coauthors (2006) lends credence to the cyclical theory. Using detailed HIV surveillance data on specific countries, they extracted the estimated natural cyclical movement of the HIV epidemic in Zimbabwe, Kenya, and Haiti and showed that in those countries, the annual number of new infections had fallen by more than plausibly could have been caused by the natural course of HIV. However, recent data from Uganda, where treatment coverage has expanded, suggest, as Alex Opio of the National AIDS Control Programme at the Ugandan Ministry of Health and others have argued, that both risk behavior and HIV prevalence rates are rising (Opio and others 2008). Thus, it is necessary to consider the discouraging possibility that Africa's incidence would stabilize at its current level, or even rise, as well as more optimistic futures in which it will continue to decline at 3 percent or more per year.

Timing and Costs of an AIDS Transition in Africa

In contrast to most other infectious diseases, HIV/AIDS spreads slowly but with seemingly inexorable momentum. The time from infection to illness is typically about eight years, with individual durations varying from five to twelve years or more. In the absence of AIDS treatment, this long lag time means that preventing an HIV infection only averts death after a median time of about eight years. Since first-line AIDS treatment postpones mortality for the median patient by four to ten years (see box 1-1), its wide availability increases the lag between HIV prevention and averted death by this same number of years. When much more expensive second-line AIDS treatment is available for patients whose first-line therapy no longer works, mortality is postponed again.

Thus, HIV-prevention programs implemented in the next few years will generate most of their mortality-reducing benefits beginning twenty years in the future. Any analysis with a shorter outlook will undervalue the effect of HIV prevention now and in the immediate future. Other policy interventions with long-term impacts include changing the uptake rate of new AIDS patients or the criteria for AIDS treatment eligibility. In this book, in an effort to capture the benefits of HIV prevention and other AIDS policies with long duration, I use a planning horizon of 2050.

Quick, Slow, or Not At All

When might an AIDS transition occur in sub-Saharan Africa? By projecting forward to the year 2050 the annual numbers of new HIV infections and AIDS deaths, one can estimate the number of years until an AIDS transition is achieved as a function of plausible rates of incidence decline and ART uptake. The three cases illustrated in figure 1-5 show differing speeds of incidence decline, from the number of new infections staying constant to a decline of 10 percent per year.[11] Each case has four possible future treatment-uptake scenarios. The uptake assumption—defined as the percentage of unmet need at the beginning of any year that is met during that year—varies from three to 80 percent.[12]

Case one (panel a) illustrates what would happen if the number of annual infections in sub-Saharan Africa remained constant at its current value of about 2 million new infections per year. With constant incidence,

FIGURE 1-5. The Timing of an African AIDS Transition at Different Rates of New Infections and Treatment

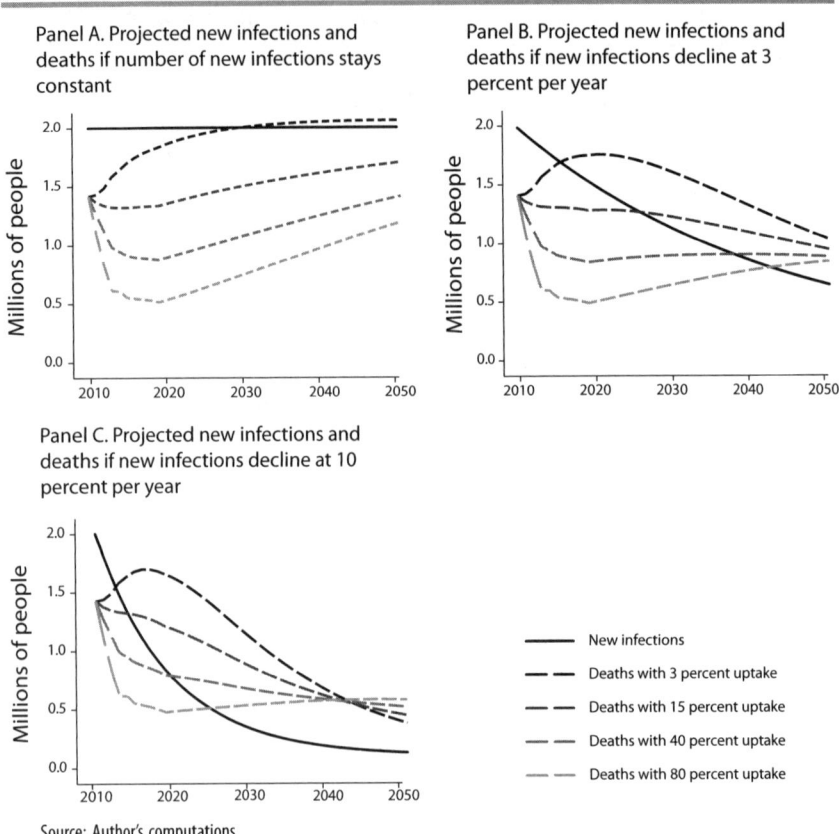

Panel A. Projected new infections and deaths if number of new infections stays constant

Panel B. Projected new infections and deaths if new infections decline at 3 percent per year

Panel C. Projected new infections and deaths if new infections decline at 10 percent per year

New infections
Deaths with 3 percent uptake
Deaths with 15 percent uptake
Deaths with 40 percent uptake
Deaths with 80 percent uptake

Source: Author's computations.

even an uptake rate of 80 percent per year would be insufficient to suppress the number of AIDS deaths beyond 2020, and more than 1 million people per year would be added to the total eventually needing treatment. At the other extreme, a policy with a 3 percent uptake rate would allow AIDS mortality to rise until it would equal the number of new cases in 2029. As a result, the explosive growth of the number of people living with HIV/AIDS would slow and then eventually reverse. But this "solution" to the problems of treatment success would reproduce for sub-Saharan Africa the breakdown described above as the first potential scenario of a failed transition. This result is akin to solving the problem of exploding population growth not with family planning, but by deliberately deploying the four horsemen of the apocalypse.

Case two reflects the more optimistic assumption that the rate of new infections continues to decline at about 3 percent per year, as it has for the last seven years (figure 1-5, panel b). But even with declining incidence, a policy that has only a 3 percent uptake rate would lead to a convergence of mortality and incidence—an outcome I define as a "transition failure" because it does not meet the condition of sustaining the reduction in AIDS mortality. But if the treatment uptake rate were 15 percent per year, AIDS mortality would remain roughly at the level successful treatment expansion achieves. Under this uptake rate, the continent would attain an AIDS transition in 2026. With more vigorous ART expansion at 40 percent or 80 percent, the AIDS transition would be attained in 2038 or 2043.

The sixteen-plus years it would take to achieve the transition in case two seems like too long to wait before turning the corner on the AIDS epidemic, especially given that decades of further expenditures on AIDS treatment would lie ahead and an uptake rate of 15 percent would leave 85 percent of patients without recourse in any year throughout this period. Case three represents what would happen with a more (perhaps excessively) optimistic 10 percent decline in the rate of new infections (panel c). With much more successful prevention and an uptake rate of 15 percent, the AIDS transition in sub-Saharan Africa could be attained in 2015. Even with much more ambitious uptake rates of 40 or 80 percent, the transition could be achieved by 2020 or 2025.

For any decline in new infections, the transition would be postponed by further expansions of access to treatment (panels b and c). Thus, while a faster rate of treatment expansion postpones death for millions, it greatly increases future costs and dependency levels. Donors and governments must carefully weigh the consequences when they expand treatment.

The AIDS Transition in Specific Country Contexts

What would AIDS transitions look like for specific countries? Table 1-2 lists selected countries for which new infections appear to have occurred more often than deaths in 2007. Assuming that each country were able to attain a 3 percent annual decline in new HIV infections—a dramatic change from past experience in every case—we can calculate the future of the epidemic under alternate plans for treatment rollout to project the implication of that plan for achieving the AIDS transition.[13]

To illustrate the projections, let Nigeria and Mozambique represent Africa and Haiti represent the worst AIDS epidemic in the Western Hemisphere. Panel a in each of the next three figures presents for each country the temporal pattern of deaths, infections, and total number of people living with HIV/AIDS, showing whether uptake is sufficient to suppress mortality and, if so, the year the AIDS transition milestone would be met. Panel b shows the number of people receiving ART and the unmet need; panel c, the future cost to the public sector (donors and government) of this time pattern of AIDS treatment; and panel d, the total cost of AIDS treatment as a proportion of projected national health spending, total health spending, and total central government spending. Each figure projects these future quantities at the approximate historical yearly uptake rate in the respective country (top row) and at a much more ambitious uptake rate of 80 percent (bottom row).[14] The incidence of new infections does not depend on the treatment uptake rate to avoid introducing additional assumptions.[15]

With an ART uptake rate of 15 percent per year, Nigeria (figure 1-6) could attain an AIDS transition by 2026 (panel a) at a cost that rises to $1.5 billion per year by 2050 (panel c) and hits a relative peak of 13 percent of its public health budget around 2018 (panel d). Mozambique (figure 1-7) could achieve a transition in 2029 with an uptake rate of 17 percent and a cost that rises to $900 million dollars and peaks relatively at 65 percent of its public health budget around 2021. Haiti (figure 1-8) has benefited greatly from the support of Paul Farmer's Partners in Health. Thanks to this assistance, the uptake is one of the highest among low-income countries, recently attaining 27.4 percent of unmet need recruited each year. At that uptake rate, the transition would occur at 2033, with costs rising to $120 million per year and peaking relatively at 12 percent of its public health budget around 2018.

But the prospect that Haiti will divert up to 12 percent of its public health budget to AIDS treatment, as is necessary for an AIDS transition, seems dim for the next decade. I project that the share of ART in public health expenditures will decline thereafter, as it does in the other scenarios presented in this section, assuming that per capita growth in all countries in a region eventually will converge to the average per capita growth recently experienced in that region. Given Haiti's decades of stagnation, one can hope—but not readily believe—that Haiti will pursue a growth path that eventually will allow it to finance AIDS treatment out of its own pocket. Clearly the achievement of an AIDS transition will make eventual self-sufficiency easier to imagine.

An uptake rate of 80 percent—far more ambitious than the historical uptake each country has achieved in recent years—would dramatically reduce AIDS deaths from now to 2050. For example, in Nigeria, the higher uptake rate would postpone almost 100,000 deaths a year by 2020, but those extra postponed deaths would cost billions of dollars that could be spent elsewhere in the economy and also would delay the AIDS transition by 17 years. Mozambique will find it extremely challenging to finance ART for the million people who would receive it under a continuation of its 17 percent rate of uptake; an 80 percent uptake rate would extend ART to 2.5 million people, but it would quickly exceed the country's total public health budget. In Haiti, the number of people dependent on AIDS treatment for survival would rise to about 200,000 by 2050 compared to 120,000 under the policy that continues the existing uptake rate. The cost burden in the year 2050 also would be 50 percent higher at $180 million a year instead of $120 million. The extra expenditure would avert about 3,000 deaths per year.

How to Make the Money Go Further

How much would an AIDS transition in sub-Saharan Africa cost? A model that allows a look at many possible scenarios helps answer this question. Critical model assumptions include a 2050 projection horizon, which captures most benefits of prevention occurring in the next decade, and a conventional social discount rate of 3 percent.[16] The future fiscal burden of a government or donor commitment to any given level of recruitment is estimated by assumptions about the unit cost of treatment in each country, the potential economies of scale as treatment numbers expand, the success rate of treatment, the proportion of patients moving from first- to second-line treatment, and other determinants. External donors bear most of these costs, except in a few middle-income countries, such as South Africa and Botswana, where the governments bear a substantial share.

The cost of an AIDS transition in sub-Saharan Africa depends on the uptake rate. A zero percent uptake rate would mean that those underwriting the treatment subsidies respect the entitlement of patients who have started subsidized treatment up to the present but assume no financial responsibility for additional patients.[17] Using available data on the mortality of AIDS patients on treatment and assuming that second-line treatment rises to 95 percent coverage of the recruited patients who fail first-line treatment by the year 2020, about half of the 3.4 million patients currently on subsidized treatment in sub-Saharan Africa will still be alive in 2050, two-thirds of whom will be on second-line therapy. As figure 1-9 shows, the annual cost of this existing cohort starts at $2.5 billion in 2010, rises to $3.3 billion in 2028 as more patients switch to second-line therapy, then declines to $2.5 billion again in 2050 as mortality thins out the number of patients at the end of the projection period. Cumulating this annual cost over the forty years at a 3 percent discount rate yields a total present value (or

FIGURE 1-6. Nigeria: Characteristics of an AIDS Transition at 15 Percent Uptake and 80 Percent Uptake of Antiretroviral Therapy (ART)

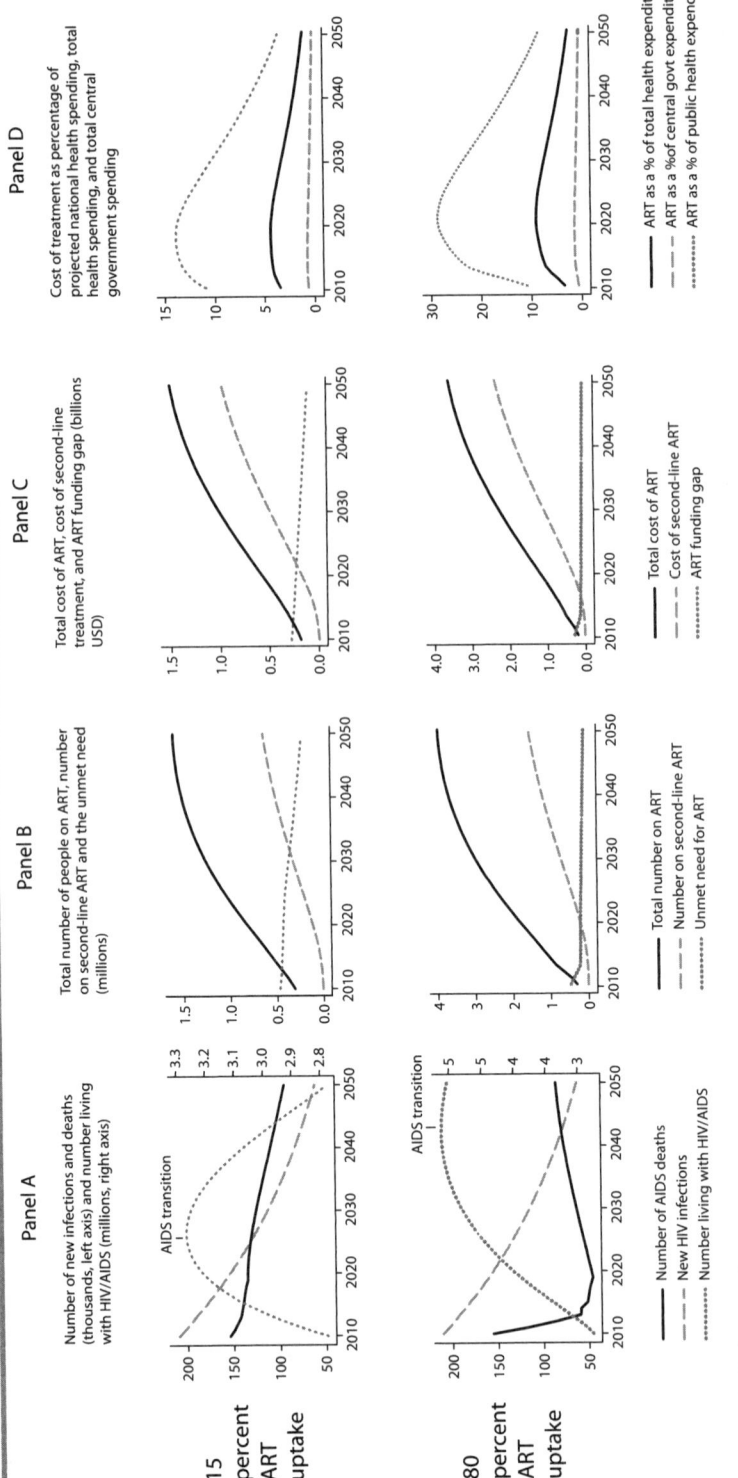

Source: Author's computations.

FIGURE 1-7. Mozambique: Characteristics of an AIDS Transition at 17 Percent Uptake and 80 Percent Uptake of Antiretroviral Therapy (ART)

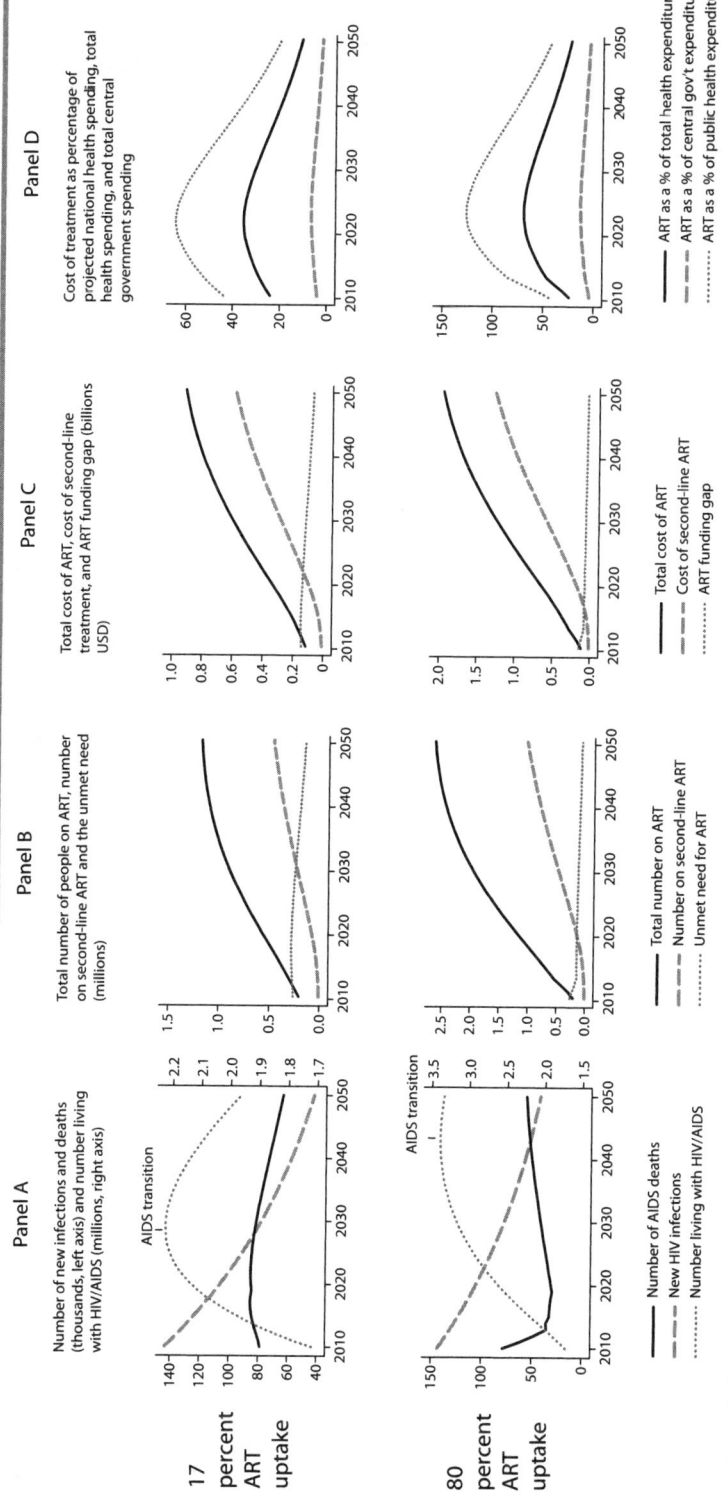

Source: Author's computations.

FIGURE 1-8. Haiti: Characteristics of an AIDS Transition at 27.4 Percent Uptake and 80 Percent Uptake of Antiretroviral Therapy (ART)

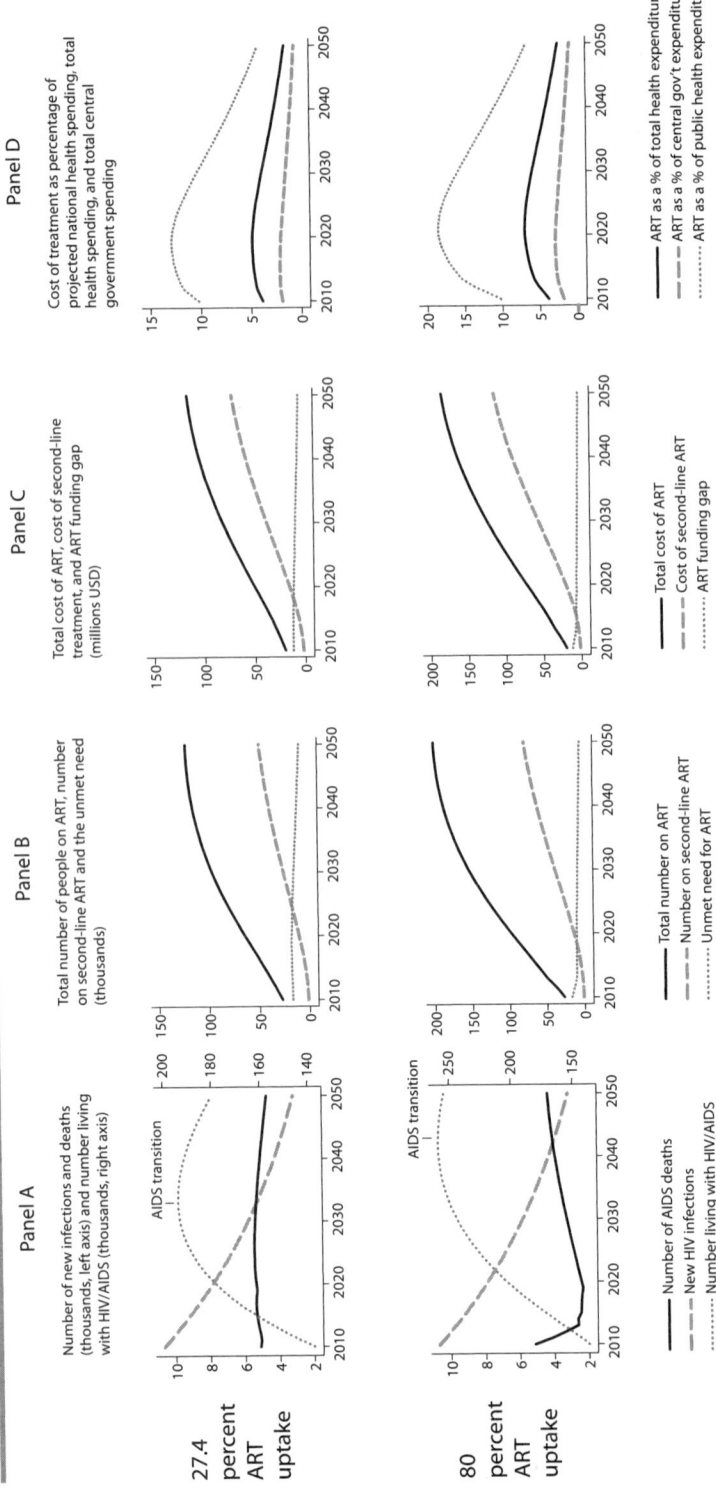

Source: Author's computations. Projections are based on the author's AIDSCost model, described in appendix C. Instructions to download and operate the program are available at www.cgdev.org/aidscost.

FIGURE 1-9. Projected Annual Costs of Antiretroviral Therapy (ART) in Sub-Saharan Africa, 2010–50

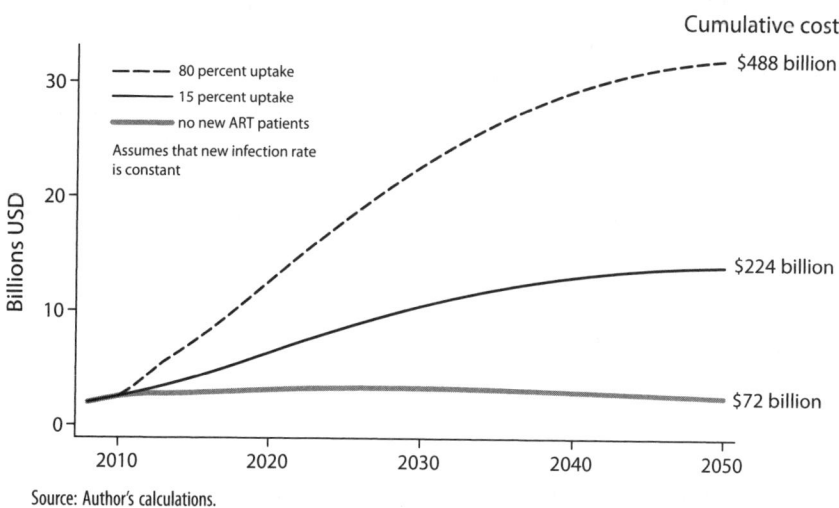

Source: Author's calculations.

endowment equivalent) of $72 billion 2009 dollars.[18] At a 3 percent interest rate, the annualized cost of this commitment would be $3 billion per year, which the international community approximately spent to subsidize AIDS treatment in low-income countries in 2009.[19]

Since a complete cessation of treatment recruitment seems unlikely and would allow AIDS mortality to rise—thus constituting a failure of the AIDS transition—figure 1-9 presents the timeline of costs for two other scenarios, each of which is defined by a constant uptake percentage. The middle line presents the future cost stream associated with funders' commitment to continue recruiting 15 percent of those needing treatment, the rate at which the average sub-Saharan country recruited patients from 2006 to 2007.[20] Because a few African countries have done much better than that, while most have done worse, a commitment to this objective might entail reallocating treatment subsidies away from countries that have recruited higher percentages to those that have done worse. Under this recruitment policy, and assuming that HIV incidence remains unchanged, figure 1-9 shows that annual treatment costs for the continent would rise from $3.3 billion now to about $12 billion by the year 2050. The total present value of the commitment would be $224 billion.[21] At a 3 percent interest rate, the annualized cost of this commitment would be $10 billion per year, about three times the international community's spending on treatment in 2009.

A much more generous commitment to provide subsidized treatment for 80 percent of those who need it each year would near the humanitarian ideal of universal coverage for AIDS treatment. Under the same assumptions as before regarding treatment success, HIV incidence, and passage to second-line treatment—but allowing for some economies of scale as treatment numbers rise in individual countries—the annual cost of this commitment would rise above $30 billion in the year 2050. The total present value of the forty-year commitment would be $488 billion.[22] At a 3 percent interest rate, the annualized cost of this commitment would be $21 billion per year, which is about seven times more than the international community spent on treatment in 2009.

Lowering Costs through Prevention

Better prevention that helps bring down the rate of new infections will reduce the cost of achieving an AIDS transition. Figure 1-10 shows that the total forty-year cost to donors and governments depends not only on commitments to patient enrollment (higher uptake rates), but also on the rate of incidence. The total present value of uptake commitments in the zero to 80 percent range is extremely sensitive to the effectiveness of HIV prevention on the continent. For example, if the annual number of new HIV infections in Africa remains unchanged at about 2 million per year, an 80 percent uptake costs a total of $488 billion (see point 1 in figure 1-10). However, with the same ambitious uptake rate, if incidence declines at 3 percent per year, costs drop to $439 billion per year, saving $49 billion over forty years, or $2.1 billion a year (see point 2). We know from panel b of figure 1-5 that the same combination of 80 percent uptake and 3 percent decline in incidence would lead to an AIDS transition in 2043; it not only saves $49 billion, but also gets Africa to an AIDS transition.

If incidence falls by 10 percent per year, the savings at an 80 percent uptake amount to $113 billion ($488 billion minus $375 billion), bringing the annualized cost of nearly universal coverage down from $21 billion to $16.1 billion per year. With this rapid rate of incidence reduction, even with an uptake rate of 80 percent, Africa would get to an AIDS transition 18 years earlier than if incidence remained at current levels, in 2025.

By contrast, consider a pessimistic case in which the number of new cases rises by 3 percent per year. The endowment equivalent of the costs over forty years for an 80 percent uptake scenario rises to $568 billion, $80 billion more than if incidence remains constant and $193 billion more than if incidence declines by 10 percent over the period. Moreover, the AIDS transition will have failed.

FIGURE 1-10. Total Forty-Year AIDS Treatment Costs in Africa by Treatment Uptake Rate and Incidence Rate, 2010–50

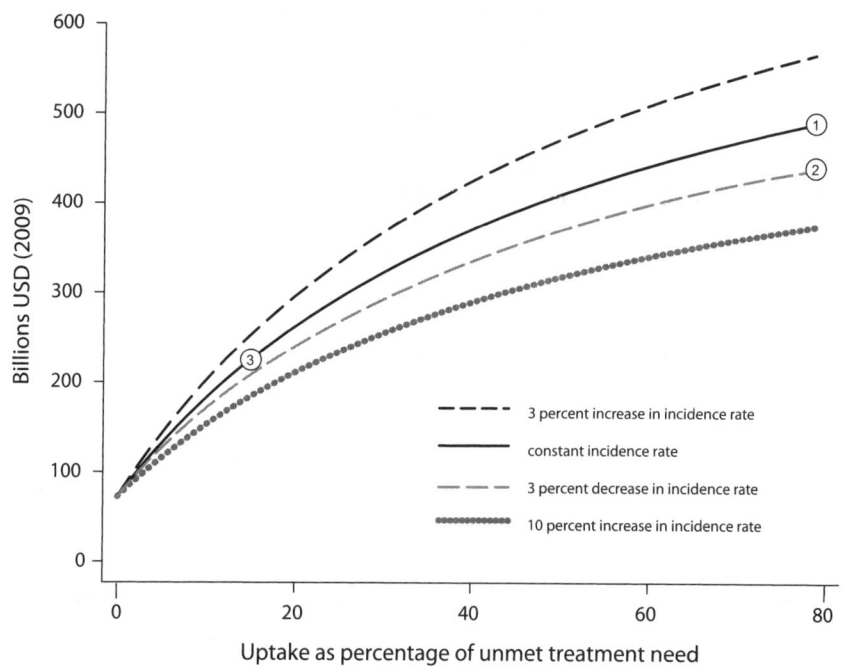

Billions USD (2009)

Uptake as percentage of unmet treatment need

3 percent increase in incidence rate

constant incidence rate

3 percent decrease in incidence rate

10 percent increase in incidence rate

Note: Future costs discounted at 3 percent

Source: Author's calculations.

Given that prodigious donor effort has been able to achieve no more than a 40 percent uptake rate for the sub-Saharan African region and now seems to be declining, it is worthwhile to focus on more affordable uptake rates. Suppose the financiers of AIDS treatment subsidies in Africa commit to meeting 15 percent of unmet treatment needed each year for the next 40 years, where "need" is defined as those having a CD4 count of less than 200.[23] At constant incidence, this commitment amounts to an endowment-equivalent commitment of $225 billion (point 3 in figure 1-10). The same commitment costs only $200 billion if the number of new HIV cases declines at 3 percent per year and only $182 billion if it declines at 10 percent per year. On the other hand, if incidence increases by 3 percent per year, the total cost of this commitment is $252 billion.

These calculations underscore how a commitment to finance a given percentage of need defines an underwriter's financial stake in HIV-prevention outcomes. The vertical distance between the upward sloping lines in fig-ure 1-10 represents the impact of future prevention success on the forty-year cost of treatment. This vertical distance widens with higher uptake commit-ments. At an uptake rate of zero, funders have no stake in future prevention success. The larger the share of future need that underwriters commit to funding, the larger will be their stake in future prevention effectiveness.

Rethinking AIDS Assistance to Facilitate an AIDS Transition

Now that the growth of HIV/AIDS funding seems to be slowing, it is a pro-pitious time for the global community to adopt an objective that sets an upper bound on future funding and improves the incentives for prevention. The goal of the AIDS transition would fill that role, but how likely is the global community to incorporate this objective into foreign aid policies? The good news is that numerous trends in today's global HIV/AIDS policy environment should facilitate this endeavor. These include:

—increasing international impatience with poor HIV-prevention per-formance excused by issues of stigma or cultural barriers;

—increasing recognition that donor support of AIDS treatment in low-income countries constitutes an expensive international entitlement from which donors and governments can only withdraw over the long term by ensuring HIV prevention (Lyman and Wittels 2010);

—increasing acceptance by donors that the eventual social development of the poorest countries depends on a long-term commitment to support their education- and health-sector achievements at levels consistent with an international humanitarian standard (as represented, for example, by the Millennium Development Goals);

—increasing acceptance by donors and recipient countries that taxpayer and philanthropic support for social services in low-income countries will depend on transparent measurement of the results these services are in-tended to deliver (Evaluation Gap Working Group 2006);

—better technology for measuring the incidence of new HIV infections at the population level;

—recognition by the international AIDS community that male circumci-sion is not only effective at reducing a man's risk of infection but also may be acceptable among adult male populations in Africa; and

—tentative acceptance by the international AIDS community that behavioral HIV prevention can be effective, although the "best practices" are highly context specific and thus must be developed and tested afresh in each national context.

The challenge for the international health community is now to build on these trends to design a new AIDS transition strategy. The key to that strategy will be to leverage the political and economic support for providing ART to the largest possible number of patients. This will ensure not only sustained support for continued uptake of new ART patients at least at the global rate of 15 percent of unmet need each year, but also a dramatic deceleration in the rate of new HIV infections.

Changing Policy at Every Level

The AIDS transition paradigm introduces an objective for each donor and national HIV/AIDS program. Programs will not be deemed successful unless they simultaneously suppress AIDS mortality and reduce the growth rate of the HIV/AIDS population. This objective will change assistance policy and practice at every level.

At the national level, an AIDS transition objective forces donors and governments to plan for AIDS treatment expansion only at the rate that evidence-based prevention programs demonstrate success in reducing incidence. The AIDS transition objective generates a demand for improved HIV-incidence measurement that will immediately expand the resources devoted to this essential task. Over the medium term, it will elicit entrepreneurial energy and biological breakthroughs to improve the technology for incidence measurement. To the extent that AIDS treatment can be shown to directly reduce HIV incidence in a given country, the scope for AIDS treatment will be expanded. But hard data must demonstrate such claims, not just mathematical models or self-reported behavioral change.

At the sub-national level, an AIDS transition objective involves local policymakers, who will be asked to show how existing HIV/AIDS treatment programs can be leveraged to improve prevention. For example, treatment programs can be required to form either an HIV-prevention arm that extends to the local community of uninfected people or a partnership with an agency specialized in results-based HIV prevention in such a population. Since budgetary constraints for supporting AIDS patients are typically national, there is scope for "trade" in AIDS treatment slots, so that sub-national districts, provinces, or programs that effectively demonstrate prevention success can give allotted treatment slots to less successful regions—perhaps in return for additional support for their malaria or maternal mortality programs. Such an internal "market" would reallocate resources to treatment and prevention efforts that effectively reduce incidence until the AIDS transition objective is satisfied.[24]

At the level of the individual patient receiving subsidized ART, those healthy enough to return to the labor force can be asked to contribute one day a month to HIV prevention in their community. Treatment programs can require patients to be members of support groups that function not only to help the patient adhere to the ART regime and regain or sustain good health as is currently done in many locales, but also to design and implement evidence-based HIV-prevention programs in local communities.

People suffering from AIDS and their advocates may object to the AIDS transition paradigm because it conditions some AIDS treatment expenditures on measured prevention success, thereby holding AIDS patients hostage to the performance of HIV-prevention programs and ultimately to the risk behavior in the community. The morality of this argument would be somewhat more compelling if financial and human resources were sufficient to treat an unlimited number of patients. However, with budget shortfalls and belt-tightening everywhere in the current environment, AIDS treatment resources will be rationed whether we like it or not. Without incidence declines, rationing will be even more severe in the future than in the present. More than ever before, AIDS treatment programs are being asked to demonstrate their efficiency. AIDS treatment advocates can increase the resources allocated to AIDS treatment if they concede the need to ensure a net decline in people living with HIV/AIDS and work actively to measure and publicize their progress toward this objective.

How PEPFAR Fits In

The 2008 reauthorization bill for PEPFAR contains an example of exactly this kind of bargain in the form of a requirement on the program. The bill mandates that the program annually report the unit costs of AIDS treatment over time. It further specifies that the number of people on treatment must be increased commensurate with the decline in the unit cost of treatment, so that the authorized treatment budget can be spread over more and more patients. This may be the first time in history that any government has mandated performance targets based on estimates of the unit costs of meeting those targets.[25]

Because U.S. authorization legislation sets an upper limit on the amount that subsequent appropriation bills can allocate to a program, the bill's authors were constrained to seek efficiency through unit cost reductions. The language of the bill gives AIDS treatment advocates an incentive to innovate in the management of treatment delivery systems in search of lower unit costs.

An alternative procedure more in keeping with the AIDS transition objective is for a donor to "authorize" its agents not only to continue to treat current patients, but also to recruit a specified share of all those who need treatment in each future year through, for example, 2050. To this end, in its December 2009 strategy document, the United States committed to expanding the number of AIDS patients who will receive U.S.-funded ART from 2.4 million to at least 4 million patients by 2014. At the same time, it promised to put greater emphasis on HIV prevention and, specifically, to prevent 12 million infections.[26]

However, it would have been preferable to make the treatment commitment in the form of a specific percentage share of treatment need rather than as a specific number of patients, so the donor and its agents could share not only the burden of future patients but also the fiscal saving from effective prevention.[27] Once it becomes apparent that the donor shares the gains from effective prevention, the donor can offer the recipient government an intertemporal trade. Under the specified assumptions on unit costs and the incidence of new infections, the future stream of these treatment costs can be estimated. For sub-Saharan Africa, the total cost of that commitment will be a great deal less if HIV incidence is reduced, as shown in figure 1-10, panels a and b. This reduction will save resources in the future, but those resources are not currently available to expand treatment rolls. A valuable role for donors is to solve this time-inconsistency problem by making a contract with the recipient country. As the recipient country presents hard evidence that HIV incidence is declining, it immediately can use a portion of the present value of the consequent savings in treatment costs to increase the current expansion of treatment access.

In the U.S. case, Congress can mandate an increase in the uptake of new patients that will hold constant the U.S. total long-term financial commitment to treatment. Such a mandate would force PEPFAR and recipient governments to measure incidence much more rigorously than they have yet done, and it also would channel political pressure for faster ART uptake toward achieving measurable reductions of HIV incidence on the ground in developing countries.

The troublesome aspect of the new PEPFAR strategy is that treatment and prevention objectives are separate. PEPFAR agents—who number in the thousands and range from in-country program staff and civil servants to contractors and NGOs—typically work on either treatment or prevention, but not on both. As a result, no one checks to see if prevention effort and success are sufficient to eventually offset the addition of more patients to the treatment rolls. It is true that both prevention and treatment would contribute to the achievement of the AIDS transition. But by failing to link them, the United States and other donors like the Global Fund to Fight AIDS, Tuberculosis and Malaria have missed a strategic opportunity to structure their AIDS assistance in a way that would more effectively motivate their agents to work toward an AIDS transition, thereby advancing the day when AIDS is a relatively rare and manageable chronic disease.

CHAPTER 2

Using Incentives to Prevent HIV Infections

As defined in the previous chapter, an AIDS transition requires maintaining recent reductions in AIDS mortality and reducing new infections even more. The last ten years have demonstrated that through concerted effort, donors and governments have reduced AIDS mortality dramatically. Unfortunately, the worldwide annual number of new infections seemingly has plateaued. While new infections appear to be declining in some countries or parts of countries, they appear to be rising in others. Thus, the most challenging aspect of the AIDS transition is HIV prevention.

The first section of this chapter reviews the evidence on the cost-effectiveness of HIV-prevention methods. Despite the surprising weakness of the available research, I conclude that HIV prevention can work provided the critical actors have the proper incentives. In the second section, I explore the degree to which performance-based incentives (PBIs) would strengthen the measurement of achievements, and I discuss the achievements themselves. I then describe six promising prevention interventions that a PBI reward structure could improve. In the third section, I propose a new approach to HIV prevention—cash on delivery (COD)—that would give local champions of developing-country HIV prevention the means to recruit allies within their own governments and civil societies to finally make headway in stemming the flow of new infections.

With Appropriate Incentives, HIV Prevention Can Work

It is depressing and even scandalous that after almost thirty years of donor-funded HIV-prevention efforts, researchers have conducted very few rigorous evaluations of these interventions (Wegbreit and others 2006; Bertozzi, Padian, and Martz 2010). Of the scant rigorous evaluations that exist, some look only at the costs or only at the health effects of an intervention, while the best guidance for resource allocation comes from those that compare the effects to the costs—known as cost-effectiveness studies. Such studies estimate the costs per unit of health benefit obtained. Costs typically are measured in dollars, and health benefits are measured either in number of HIV cases averted or in years of additional healthy life, which can be quantified as "disability-adjusted life years" (DALYs) gained.[1]

Recognizing that health service costs depend heavily on the cost of labor and other locally purchased inputs that vary dramatically by a country's per capita GDP, a useful convention is to express the dollar cost per additional DALY gained as a proportion of the per capita GDP of the country in which the intervention has been performed. A recent review of cost-effectiveness studies reports,

> "First, all HIV-prevention interventions reviewed here are highly cost effective; that is, the cost per DALY is far less than [the dollar value of] GDP per capita; and most interventions in Africa cost less than 30% of [the dollar value of] GDP per capita and 40% in other regions. Second, all HIV-prevention interventions reviewed are cost effective when compared to other life saving interventions including HIV treatment, which is consistent with other recent comparative results" (Galarraga and others 2009, p. 8).

Among the interventions that different studies find to be cost-effective are male circumcision, sex education classes in schools (Hogan and others 2005), and a system of rewards for safe behavior and legal sanctions for risky behavior for prostitutes in the Dominican Republic (Sweat, Kerrigan, and others 2006).

Unfortunately, few of these favorable cost-effectiveness findings on HIV prevention are supported by the most rigorous kind of evidence, known as randomized controlled trials. What exactly is a randomized controlled trial? To begin with, evaluation experts define the health benefit from an intervention as the difference between the health status of people who have received the intervention and the best estimate of what their health status would have been without the intervention. They apply the term "counterfactual" to the estimated health status of these same people without the intervention because it refers to a situation that did not actually occur. For an evaluation study to provide the most reliable guidance to decisionmakers, its estimate of the intervention's benefit must be computed as the improvement with respect to a rigorously estimated counterfactual. Experts widely agree that the most reliable and rigorous method for estimating the counterfactual, and thus for calculating the improvement caused by the intervention, is to use a randomized controlled trial (Evaluation Gap Working Group 2006).

What do the randomized controlled trials that have been carried out on HIV prevention show? Among the thirty-seven distinct trials of thirty-nine interventions to reduce HIV infection, only five have found a benefit (Padian and others 2010). Of these, three have produced strong evidence that adult male circumcision reduces the man's chance of infection by somewhere between 33 to 68 percent, one shows promise for a vaccine, and one, which finds HIV-prevention benefits to treating curable sexually transmitted infection (STI), is contradicted by other equally rigorous experiments.[2] Promising interventions that have failed to show benefits in randomized controlled trials include vaginal microbicide (twelve);[3] behavioral interventions using counseling, education, and condom distribution (seven); microfinance (one); the diaphragm (one); and antiretroviral pills taken to prevent infection from a risky contact (one).

Some conclude from these discouraging results that HIV prevention is a hopeless task. But I believe evidence is ample that HIV prevention can and will achieve much greater success in the next ten years than it has in the last thirty. The failures of these randomized controlled trials to convincingly reduce HIV incidence do not constitute proof that these interventions do not work. Box 2-1 explores several reasons these tests can fail to measure the true impact of intervention. Most notably, to meet the requirements imposed by ethics review boards, the researchers in almost all HIV-prevention trials were—and still are—required to provide substantial HIV-prevention interventions to those not receiving the tested intervention, impeding the proper measurement of prevention efforts.

For example, consider the test of diaphragm use for HIV prevention. The subjects were randomly allocated to either a control group that did not receive a diaphragm or an experimental group that did. The idea was to test whether the rate of new HIV infections would be smaller among patients in the experimental group than among those in the control group. However, the ethics review boards felt that it would be unethical to withhold all HIV prevention from the women who would not receive a

---

BOX 2-1. Can Ethics "Blind" Attempts to Learn How Well Prevention Works?

Although randomized controlled trials (RCTs) have the best chance of any evaluation method at giving an accurate estimate of the health improvement due to an intervention, they still can fail to discover the true impact of a valuable intervention for several reasons. First, the test may be underpowered: for lack of foresight or resources, the researchers collect samples so small that the natural variation across intervention sites is large enough to hide the true average benefit in the average site. Second, an intervention might not work in the particular context in which it is tested, yet it could work elsewhere. Third, the mere fact that people in the control group know they are being studied might induce them to behave safely, the so-called Hawthorne effect. And fourth, to meet the requirements imposed by ethical review boards, the researchers in almost all HIV-prevention trials are required to provide substantial HIV-prevention interventions to those not receiving the tested intervention—in effect impeding the proper measurement of prevention efforts (see Padian and others 2010).

The figure here shows how ethical constraints might hide success. The vertical axis measures how many new HIV infections, measured as the percentage of the baseline observation, might be observed during the year after the beginning of the trial of a new prevention intervention in four hypothetical groups of randomly allocated villages. The people in the first group of villages receive the standard of care in the national context; the only additional benefit from the study that they might receive is from information circulating in the community from the media and word-of-mouth, perhaps augmented by national information and prevention campaigns. In the hypothetical example, the number of new cases in this group declines by 5 percent (from 100 to 95) on average. The error bars extending above and below show the range of variation across the villages in the group. Typically ethical boards forbid an RCT from collecting data on this group of villages on the grounds that it would be unethical to have any contact with them without offering them prevention interventions.

The second bar shows a hypothetical 30 percent average reduction in incidence in the group of villages that receives a package of interventions mandated by the RCT's ethics panel for everyone contacted

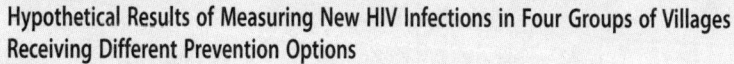

Hypothetical Results of Measuring New HIV Infections in Four Groups of Villages Receiving Different Prevention Options

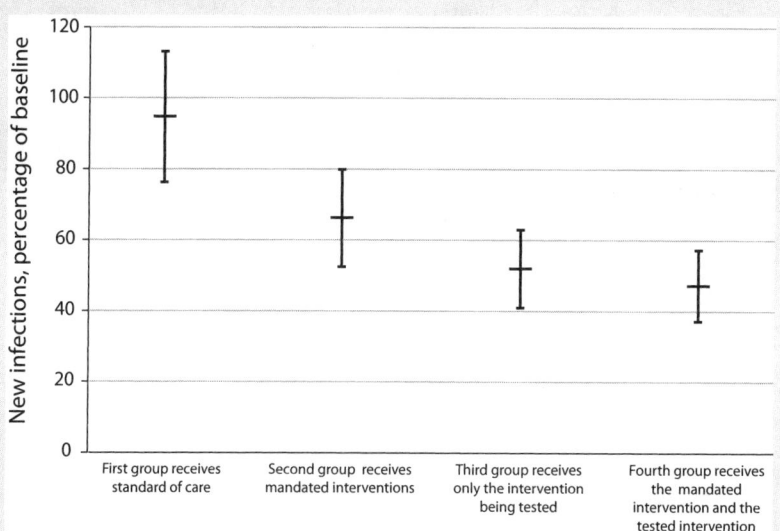

Source: Author's construction

by the RCT. The interventions in this group might include intensive counseling about the dangers of HIV infection and conventional methods of protection—such as partner reduction and condom use—and they might also include condom distribution and diagnosis and treatment of the curable sexually transmitted infections (see Padian and others 2010). This group is considered to be the control group for the RCT even though it receives some benefit, albeit not from the intervention being tested.

Suppose a third group of villages receives only the intervention being tested. Such an intervention would be prohibited by the ethical requirement that all contacted villages receive the mandated intervention package, but it alone could result in an incidence rate that is on average 45 percent lower than the standard-of-care villages.

The fourth group of villages receives both the mandated intervention package and the intervention being tested. In this hypothetical example, the fourth group experiences the most benefit, with the

(continued)

average village having an incidence fully 50 percent lower than it would have been without the package of interventions.

Even though the tested intervention alone would show a remarkable improvement over the standard of care, an RCT that is allowed to collect data only on the second and fourth groups of villages will fail to find a statistically significant benefit of the tested intervention. Statistical analysis will show that despite the difference in the average incidence between the second and fourth groups, the variation around the averages in the two groups (shown by the overlapping error bars) means that the difference in the averages might be due only to chance.

Despite the rigor of the methods, this hypothetical RCT reaches a false conclusion. If the researchers had been able to compare either group that includes the intervention being tested to the villages receiving only the local standard of care, they would have found that prevention works. Because they have been "blinded" by ethical constraints, they have not been able to measure the true benefits of the interventions.

diaphragm. They insisted that the researchers provide these women with condom promotion, enhanced diagnosis and treatment of curable STIs (like gonorrhea, syphilis, and chlamydia), and risk-reduction counseling (see table 2-1). Thus, instead of comparing the effectiveness of the diaphragm to the effectiveness of any actions that women in the study area were taking without intervention, the researchers were obliged to compare the effectiveness of the diaphragm to a package of interventions generally thought to be among the most effective. If the package was sufficiently effective at preventing HIV, the addition of a diaphragm would have lacked any room to make any difference.

The conditions that the ethics review boards placed on the diaphragm experiment are typical for prevention studies. As a result, evidence that prevention works might be lacking because the tested interventions, although intrinsically quite useful, have not been sufficiently better than the package of services provided to the control group (Lagakos and Gable 2008). Many informal study reports that risk behavior or HIV incidence improved in the control group support the possibility that all these interventions work. Rigorously establishing this conclusion through better

Table 2-1. Components of Prevention Services Offered to Control Groups in Thirty-Six Randomized Controlled Trials for HIV Prevention

| | *Number of trials with prevention services in control groups* | | | |
Type of intervention	*Number of trials*	*Risk reduction counseling/ education*	*Condom promotion*	*Enhanced services for sexually transmitted infections*
Behavioral (including risk reduction counseling and condom promotion)	7	5	4	1
Diaphragm	1	1	1	1
Microbicides	12	12	12	12
Pre-exposure prophylaxis[a]	1	1	1	0
Male circumcision	4	4	4	4
Treatment of curable sexually transmitted infections	9	7	8	6
Vaccines	4	4	3	2
Total	38	34 (89%)	33 (87%)	26 (68%)

Source: Personal communication with Sandi McCoy and Nancy Padian of the University of California, San Francisco, February 15, 2010, based on Padian and others 2010.

a. This intervention consists of providing antiretroviral medication to uninfected people prior to their exposure, for example, through unprotected sex or needle sharing.

study design would greatly advance HIV-prevention science and policy. Meanwhile, informal reports and decreased infection rates in Thailand, Uganda, and other countries encourage the world to find ways to improve prevention.

Using Performance-Based Incentives for HIV Prevention

How can the most promising existing interventions be scaled up, and what will best motivate the implementers? Part of the answer may lie in a relatively new policy instrument for the health sector—the application of performance-based incentives to increase the productivity or improve the quality of health care. What exactly are PBIs? Rena Eichler and Ruth Levine, authors of *Performance Incentives for Global Health*, define them as "the transfer of money or material goods conditional on taking a measurable action or achieving a predetermined performance target." They include "incentives on both the demand and the supply sides, at both individual and collective levels, [which operate at] the interface between provider and patient." But they exclude "the conditional payments that donor agencies offer to national [or sub-national] governments" (Eichler, Levine, and Performance-Based Incentives Working Group 2009, p. 6).[4]

The purpose of PBIs is to adjust individual agents' incentives to better align with the interests of the communities and the countries they are servicing. On the demand side, PBIs should heighten the interest of individual clients. On the supply side, they should motivate service providers to exert more effort toward program objectives. Whether they can improve day-to-day HIV-prevention operations or AIDS treatment remains to be explored sufficiently—so far, they have undergone little rigorous evaluation—but results from studies reviewed by Eichler, Levine, and Performance-Based Incentives Working Group (2009) are promising.

In rural Malawi, for example, University of Michigan researcher Rebecca Thornton studied a demand-side PBI by randomizing the distribution to clients of vouchers worth up to a day's wage, redeemable on submission to an HIV test and receipt of the results at a nearby voluntary counseling and testing clinic. She found that while demand for HIV testing was substantial even in the absence of a cash incentive, any positive amount nearly doubled uptake of HIV testing. She also found that HIV-positive respondents who learned their test results were significantly more likely to purchase condoms in follow-up interviews (Thornton 2008).[5]

Also in Malawi, George Washington University assistant professor of global health Sarah Baird and others (2010) randomized a conditional cash transfer that sought to estimate the effect of receiving a small cash payment of $15 or less to girls and their families conditional on girls' school attendance.[6] Some girls received the cash regardless of whether they went to school, others only if they went to school, and others received nothing. The authors found that one year after the intervention, cash transfers led to increases in self-reported school attendance and declines in early marriage, pregnancy, sexual activity, risky sexual behavior, and coital frequency for the sexually active. Girls who received cash were more likely to attend school regardless of whether the cash was conditional on attendance. Furthermore, at the end of eighteen months, the percentage of HIV infection among the girls who had received the cash was 1.2 percent, compared to 3 percent among those who had not. In other words, a monthly payment of no more than $15 seems to have achieved a 60 percent reduction in HIV infection. To explain how cash and improved school attendance might have reduced the girls' sexual activity, the authors suggest that school attendance made the girls less available for sexual liaisons or the cash transfer possibly relieved girls of the need to trade sex for school expenses. Particularly indicative was the finding that only 2 percent of the girls who received cash had partners 25 years or older, compared to 21 percent of the girls who had not received money. The authors caution that a longer study would be required to estimate how long the benefits persist (Baird and others 2010).

Conditional cash transfers also might more directly link to HIV prevention. Since the same sexually risky behavior that transmits HIV also transmits diseases such as genital herpes, gonorrhea, and syphilis, people who protect from these less dangerous, curable STIs also are protecting from HIV. Carol Medlin and Damien de Walque (2008), currently at the Bill and Melinda Gates Foundation and the World Bank, respectively, suggest that paying program participants for remaining free of curable STI infections might be a practical observable proxy for risky sexual behavior on which to condition cash transfers. By conditioning the transfer on a reversible event (an STI infection), instead of an irreversible one (an HIV infection), such a conditional transfer program can continue to provide rewards for safe behavior to people who have previously failed the condition, a group of particular interest for curbing the epidemic. Furthermore, HIV-positive people can continue to receive rewards for safe behavior, for which they would be forever ineligible if the condition were HIV-negative status.

UC Berkeley health economist William Dow, Damien de Walque, and Rose Nathan of the Ifakara Health Institute have applied this lesson by designing just such a randomized controlled trial in Tanzania.[7] Of the young adults who were offered a cash payment for remaining free of a curable sexually transmitted infection, only 9 percent became infected after a year, compared to 12 percent of those not offered the incentive. The result was a 25 percent reduction in infection. The study was not large or long enough to test whether the payment reduced HIV infection. A planned resurvey of participants a year after the conditional transfers have ended will reveal whether the benefits persist.

Incentives such as these are urgently needed to energize the following six neglected but promising HIV/AIDS-prevention strategies:

—improved targeting of HIV prevention in HIV "hot spots";

—expansion of access to male circumcision;

—integration of family planning services into HIV testing and AIDS treatment facilities;

—reorientation of HIV testing toward in-home services for couples, partially as a substitute for facility-based testing of individuals;

—use of AIDS treatment to suppress transmission to existing partners; and

—mobilization of donor-funded AIDS patients for HIV prevention.

Incentives to Target HIV Hot Spots

The first step in a successful prevention campaign is to gather the epidemiological data to discern where and among whom HIV infections are spreading most rapidly. Two mathematicians made the epidemiological case for controlling STIs among high-risk populations as a matter of public health with mathematical rigor 35 years ago (Hethecote and Yorke 1984). The World Bank and other organizations began to argue for prioritizing high-risk groups in the next decade (Ainsworth and Over 1997), but program administrators believed that population-wide approaches would be more effective and less stigmatizing. Beginning in about 2007, however, UNAIDS, the Joint United Nations Program on HIV/AIDS, embraced the new slogan "Know your epidemic—Know your response" (Wilson and Halperin 2008). Economists also support this approach because the beneficial effects of prevention among those with high risk spill over to people outside the high-risk groups (Over and Aral 2006). Recent evidence from the Avahan project in India, described in box 2-2, provides some support for these spillover effects by showing a correlation between HIV prevalence rates among female sex workers and HIV prevalence rates at antenatal clinics, which serve some of the general population (Alary and others 2010).

Economic logic supports placing the highest priority on the high-risk groups that are relatively easy to access. Figure 2-1 shows how the various groups of the population can be organized by both risk and accessibility. Governments with low coverage of all these groups can start by ensuring coverage of the groups in the northeast corner of the diagram, which might include sex workers in brothels, intravenous drug users in treatment programs, and men who have sex with men. In countries where HIV prevalence is low in the general population, virtually universal coverage of all high-risk groups might be enough to reverse the course of the epidemic and accomplish the AIDS transition. In countries with more generalized epidemics, universal coverage of all high-risk groups is necessary but insufficient; in these countries, reaching an AIDS transition requires interventions to reach out actively to the general population, in particular through widespread scale-up of male circumcision as well as couples testing and counseling.

Unfortunately, in many countries health officials do not know where to find these high-risk groups or how to contact them without intimidation. A technique called Priorities for Local AIDS Control Efforts, or the PLACE Method, was developed in the last ten years to address this problem, especially in African epidemiological contexts (Weir and others 2002; Weir,

BOX 2-2. Avahan: The India HIV-Prevention Initiative
Gina Dallabetta

In 2003 the Bill & Melinda Gates Foundation began its large HIV-prevention program, the India AIDS Initiative, later called Avahan, to curtail the spread of HIV in India. At the time, there was a sense of urgency about the rising prevalence of HIV in the world's second-most populous country. The foundation had three primary goals for this initiative: to build an HIV-prevention model at scale in India, catalyze others to take over and replicate best practices, and foster and disseminate learning within India and worldwide.

Avahan has built a successful, large-scale HIV-intervention program in its first five years. It operates in six Indian states that accounted for 83 percent of HIV infections in 2002 and have a combined population of 300 million people. At the end of the first five-year phase in March 2009 to build a model at scale, Avahan prevention programs in these states were providing prevention services to approximately 221,000 female sex workers, 82,000 high-risk men who have sex with men and transgendered people, 18,000 injecting drug users, and 5 million men who are long-distance truckers and clients of sex workers (Bill & Melinda Gates Foundation 2010). In April 2009 Avahan entered its second five-year phase, which focuses on the transition of the project to "natural owners," such as the government of India and communities it has served since the beginning of the HIV epidemic. "Avahan," or "call to action," refers to the collaborative effort of the partner organizations, hundreds of grassroots NGOs, thousands of peer educators, and others working on this initiative. The initial funding commitment for Avahan was US$250 million for the first five years, with an additional US$58 million committed in 2006.

Given the nature of India's HIV epidemic, Avahan's aim is to help slow the transmission of HIV to the general population by raising prevention coverage to 80 percent of high-risk and bridge groups across large geographic areas. Experts thought such an approach would be difficult to accomplish in India because of the scale and diversity of the country as well as the risk of further stigmatizing these groups. Given the charter, size, and anticipated complexity of

(continued)

the initiative, the foundation opened an India office and recruited local staff with a mix of for-profit and public health backgrounds. The hope was that this marriage of private-sector management skills and public health skills would be most effective at quickly rolling out such a large-scale program.

Avahan pioneered innovative approaches to the design, organization, execution, and management of a large-scale targeted HIV-prevention campaign. In the design phase, implementing partners conducted detailed mapping and size estimations of the high-risk groups across the districts. This mapping activity, which was periodically repeated and refined as the targeted groups learned to trust the implementers, became the statistical foundation for managing operations and estimating the coverage rate.

Avahan gave grants to nine lead partners, who in turn sub-granted and supported 134 grassroots NGOs, who hired and trained physicians, nurses, counselors, and about 7,500 peer outreach workers and staff supervisors to provide services. This implementation structure was supported by advocacy, capacity-building, monitoring and evaluation, and knowledge-building partners.

To support service expansion, Avahan created a set of basic technical and managerial implementation standards to guide programs and to standardize monitoring while giving the programs the flexibility to customize implementation based on local needs. To maintain focus on the expansion of prevention service delivery, the management process followed at every level included specific milestones in line with these standards; frequent and regular field visits by lead partners, capacity-building partners, and foundation staff; regular scrutiny of routine monitoring data; and regular, frequent, and formal joint progress reviews of the program and the data to take corrective action as needed. This frequent and close examination of the data resulted in many small course corrections and a few major shifts in implementation. A recent special issue of the journal *Sexually Transmitted Infections* contains several papers describing and assessing the Avahan project (for example, Alary and others 2010).

Gina Dallabetta is a senior program officer at the Bill & Melinda Gates Foundation.

FIGURE 2-1. Subjective Classification of Groups by Behavior and Accessibility

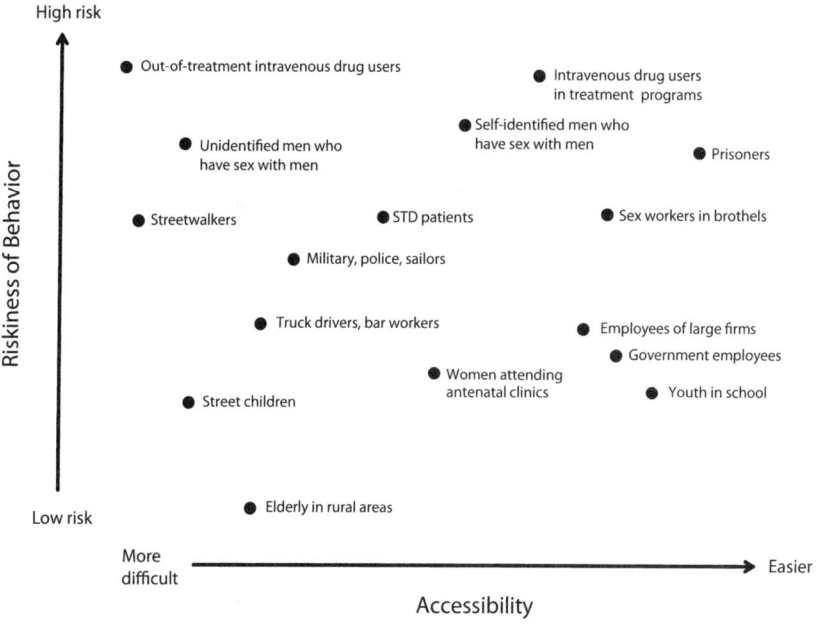

Source: Author's construction

Pailman, and others 2003; Weir, Tate, and others 2004). The method uses interviewers' contacts with taxi drivers, market women, and other people on the street to identify the "hot spots" in town, where people gather to look for a sexual liaison. Although the U.S. Agency for International Development funded the formative research to develop this technique and field test it in a dozen African cities, neither that agency nor the President's Emergency Plan for AIDS Relief (PEPFAR) has attempted to evaluate the technique using rigorous impact evaluation methods or scale up its implementation to saturate the high-risk locations in even a single city or small pilot region of any African country with prevention messages and condoms.

A variety of other techniques exist for reaching high-risk populations with needed interventions that promote and distribute condoms and train people in their effective use. Unfortunately, few of these techniques benefit from the rigorous impact evaluation that has been exercised on biomedical prevention techniques or treatment interventions (Wegbreit and others 2006; Lagakos and Gable 2008; Bertozzi, Padian, and Martz 2010). A specific need is for more rigorous evaluation than the simple correlations available from the Avahan data of the spillover benefits of targeted interventions on the nearby general populations (box 2-2 and Alary and others 2010).

Further hampering implementation of these techniques, most governments and donors have been reluctant for ideological reasons to implement these targeted HIV-prevention programs fully even in the southern cone of Africa, where the epidemic has infected a quarter of the adult population. People on the left of the political spectrum rightfully are concerned about protecting people with high-risk behavior from human-rights abuses by government or nongovernment actors. They point out that driving high-risk groups underground will make it much harder to help alter risky behavior. People on the right of the spectrum oppose providing any government interventions to groups whose behavior they reproach. Observers who know and understand the social contexts of these target populations note that only part of any given risk group is likely to fall into the high-risk, high-accessibility category represented in the top right of figure 2-1.

Critics are correct to point out that the mathematical models demonstrating the superior cost-effectiveness of interventions with high-risk groups typically assume that an intervention can accurately reach a specific risk group and change its behavior by a given amount. Claiming such accurate targeting is as unrealistic as it is for a telephone-marketing firm to assure its client that every phone call will reach a potential user of the client's product. In reality, people with high-risk behavior are dispersed among more general populations and can only be reached by going through an access channel—for example, sexually active adults at bars. Finding the best such channel, however, is difficult. To be most effective in reaching a given target group, an access channel ideally would be highly sensitive, attaining high coverage of the group, and also highly specific, reaching few people not in the group. Table 2-2 shows a hypothetical cross-tabulation of some of the epidemiologically important high-risk groups arrayed against a set of hypothetical access channels. Table entries suggest plausible degrees of the sensitivity and specificity of each access channel for each risk group.[8]

For example, suppose one would like to reach prostitutes. The proportion of all prostitutes such messages reach through mass media may be low if most prostitutes in a country are illiterate or lack access to radio or television. As a result, the mass-media access channel would have low sensitivity. In relation to the entire audience of mass media, prostitutes would be a small percentage, giving a low score on the specificity of the access channel. An intervention that operates using the PLACE method by accessing its audience through conversations in bars and dance venues would reach a high proportion of all prostitutes and thus score high on sensitivity. At the same time, it would still score low on specificity because many people thus contacted will not be prostitutes.

Real-world prevention interventions, such as the Avahan initiative in India (box 2-2), take for granted that they must pass through the appropriate channel to access their clients. However, evaluations of prevention interventions have often focused on a single channel, thus failing to provide financiers with evidence of the effectiveness of various channels or channel mixes at achieving prevention goals in a given target population. Introducing PBIs is one way to ameliorate this situation. If population-based surveys were to measure true coverage of the intended target group, PBIs could be designed at the level of the target group rather than the level of the channel. With incentives conditional on prevention programs reaching the target group, prevention agencies would be motivated to find the most effective mix of channels for reaching that group.[9] In comparison to a prevention program broadcast to the entire population, a program targeted to a specific group will typically cost more per person reached. But this higher cost is justified if targeting makes the program more effective at changing behavior.

A starting point for introducing PBIs is to delegate the job of conducting PLACE-style surveys to district and municipal governments throughout the country. A country could assemble a unified portrayal of the degree to which its HIV transmission "hot spots" are covered by prevention interventions by charging each district of the country with mapping its hot spots and reporting monthly on the proportion that are covered. National-level AIDS programming authorities could assemble these reports into nationwide maps and be held accountable for making improvements.

Incentives to Increase Male Circumcision

The evidence that male circumcision protects men from HIV infection has accumulated from observational and experimental studies. The first observational study was a cross-country regression that showed a remarkable negative association between male circumcision prevalence and HIV prevalence (Bongaarts and others 1989). But skeptics expressed doubt about a causal link because male circumcision is correlated with religious affiliation, which might be responsible for differences in HIV prevalence given religious differences in sexual mores. For example, one cross-section study of HIV prevalence did not find a correlation between infection and male circumcision after controlling for the percentage of Muslims in the population and seven other socioeconomic variables (Over 1998). Because these other variables

TABLE 2-2. Getting Out the Message: Channels to Reach Groups at Risk of Contracting HIV

		Sensitivity/specificity of access channels[a]					
Group at Risk of Contracting HIV	Size	Audience of mass media	Prisoners, soldiers, students, or workers in prisons, barracks, schools, or work sites	Sexually active adults at bars	Patients at general health care clinics	Clients and workers at family planning and sexually transmitted disease clinics	Residents of a neighborhood
From sex:							
Prostitutes	20	Low/Low	Low/Low	High/Low	Medium/Low	High/Low	Medium/Medium
Clients of prostitutes	100	Medium/Low	High/Low	High/Low	Medium/Low	High/Low	Low/Low
Sexually active adolescents	2,000	Low/Low	Medium/Low	Low/Low	Medium/Low	Medium/Low	Low/Low
Adults with multiple partners	2,000	High/Medium	High/Medium	High/High	Medium/Low	Medium/High	High/Low
From transfusions:	10,000	Medium/High	Medium/High	Low/Medium	High/High	Low/Medium	High/High
From needles:	5	High/Low	Low/Low	Medium/Low	High/Medium	High/High	Low/Low

Source: Over and Piot (1996).

a. Sensitivity is defined as the proportion of the target group reached by a message. Specificity is the proportion of those reached who are in the target group. "High" is defined as greater than two-thirds; "medium" is defined as one-third to two-thirds; "low" is defined as less than one-third.

confounded the effect of male circumcision in observational data, a randomized trial offered the best hope of determining the potential benefit of male circumcision.

In the last few years, randomized controlled trials in Uganda (Gray and others 2007), South Africa (Auvert and others 2005), and Kenya (Bailey and others 2007) have confirmed that the association between male circumcision and HIV is indeed causal. In fact, the ethics review process halted the Kenyan trial after observing that 22 of the 1,391 circumcised men became HIV infected compared to 47 among the 1,393 uncircumcised group. Because the risk of becoming infected during the trial period was 53 percent smaller for the circumcised, the researchers suggested that male circumcision is comparable to a 50 percent effective vaccination. Circumcision seemed to protect men from HIV equally well in Uganda (a 51 percent reduction in risk) and perhaps even more in South Africa (a 60 percent reduction in risk).[10] Furthermore, none of the studies found evidence that circumcised men might increase their risky behavior and thereby offset some of the advantage of the circumcision.

As the encouraging results on male circumcision have accumulated,[11] researchers have increasingly turned from the question of efficacy to those of feasibility and field-effectiveness. Small-scale non-random studies have generally supported the feasibility of scaling up male circumcision access to the general population in Africa. Building on these research results, PEPFAR should allocate a substantial portion of its discretionary resources to making clean and safe circumcision at least as easily accessible as antiretroviral therapy (ART) to the male populations in all the PEPFAR countries. It also should fund studies confirming that male circumcision is as effective in the field as it has proved in the experimental studies.

The fact that male circumcision is still somewhat controversial in some countries limits the role of both demand- and supply-side PBIs. For example, a donor-sponsored policy of offering individual men payments to accept circumcision might engender invidious charges of imperial plots against African men. On the supply side, the same considerations would prevent using PBIs to increase uptake. However, incentives could be designed to motivate providers to maintain the quality of their service (by rewarding user satisfaction) and perform efficiently (keeping waiting lines short and unit costs to a minimum).

Incentives to Integrate Family Planning with AIDS Treatment

Another key HIV-prevention strategy that has not been sufficiently deployed is family planning. While programs to prevent mother-to-child transmission of HIV are increasingly successful, they are still costly and complicated. Every child that is infected despite these efforts will be costly to treat for his or her entire life. Furthermore, despite the efficacy and increased availability of AIDS treatment, such children stand a greater-than-average chance of becoming orphans.

In view of the private and social cost incurred for each HIV-infected child, AIDS-treatment programs and family-planning programs should join forces to ensure that every HIV-positive woman has free and easy access to the birth control method of her choice, without fear of stigmatization. Unfortunately, owing to the lack of integration of family planning and AIDS treatment, unmet need for contraception appears to be substantial among HIV-positive women. As early as 1993, a study found that 60 percent of HIV-positive women would prefer not to have more children (Allen, Serufilira, Gruber, and others 1993). Other studies have found that medical intervention to prevent mother-to-child transmission of HIV once a women is pregnant is less or equally cost-effective than family planning in several studies (Stover and others 2003; Sweat and others 2004; Reynolds and others 2006). Three authors of these studies point out that the existing low levels of contraception in sub-Saharan Africa have probably prevented 173,000 HIV-infected births each recent year and that provision of family planning services to the those with unmet need can avert an additional 160,000 HIV-positive births every year (Reynolds, Steiner, and Cates 2005).

PBIs can strengthen this approach by rewarding clinics for offering family planning services to HIV-infected pregnant clients. As is the case for male circumcision, these rewards can be based on clients' satisfaction with the counseling they receive and the freedom of choice they report, rather than on uptake of family planning methods.

Incentives to Provide Couples Testing and Counseling

As a supplement to provider-initiated testing, PEPFAR and other donors should evaluate the feasibility and effectiveness of wide-scale couples counseling in the home. In a presentation at the Center for Global Development, HIV-testing researcher Susan Allen (2010) argued that the enormous expansion of HIV testing has had little beneficial impact on reducing risk behavior because it has predominantly been provided to individuals, not couples. In combination with messaging that couples should be faithful to each other, individual testing even may have accelerated the spread of the epidemic among couples who are not aware that they have different HIV test results. An explanation can be found in a brief detour through the economic theory of transactions.

One of the most influential papers ever written in economics, and the Nobel prize–winning research that followed, argues that markets function very poorly or not at all when the parties to a transaction have different amounts of information about the commodity being exchanged—the problem of "asymmetric information" (Akerlof 1970). For example, used cars are harder to sell than they should be because sellers know more about the condition of the car than do the buyers. Potential buyers anticipate being disappointed by the quality of the car they buy, and potential sellers anticipate being disappointed by the price they will be offered. As a result, car owners have less incentive to maintain their cars for eventual resale, so used cars have lower quality and sell for less, on average, than they would if both parties to all used car sales had equal, or "symmetric," information about the car under consideration.

The extension to sexual transactions is direct. Suppose two people are negotiating a sexual encounter. In the absence of couples testing, either person might know his or her own HIV status, but neither can reliably know the status of the other. Each party to a sexual transaction anticipates being disappointed by the infection status of his or her potential partner. Just as asymmetric information reduces the incentive for car owners to maintain their cars, it reduces the incentive for an individual to remain HIV negative. Furthermore, in the absence of shared information that one member of a sexual partnership is HIV positive, which would be a reason for condom use, increased fidelity within the partnership simply shortens the time until the uninfected partner will also be infected.

Thus, as long as information on HIV status is absent or asymmetric within a partnership, the advantage of fidelity is reduced. Asymmetric information discourages the formation and the survival of monogamous partnerships. Conversely, in most situations shared accurate information about each other's HIV status increases the advantage of fidelity to the partnership.[12] A certificate of HIV status that an individual could choose to show to a spouse or potential future partner is a partial solution to this problem. But such certificates would be objects of counterfeiting rings.[13] The only full solution is to offer couples counseling, a process in which members of the partnership learn their own and their partner's status from a trusted source—in the presence of a trained and experienced counselor to help them cope with the implications for their relationship of any of the possible joint-testing outcomes.

According to Allen, when counselors are trained explicitly in couples counseling and individuals seeking testing are encouraged to bring their primary sexual partners for joint testing, HIV testing does indeed work to reduce risk behavior among both discordant and concordant-negative couples. Although no randomized trials exist to support her proposition, the fact that such couples in Uganda had an infection rate of 12 percent when they were not jointly tested (Quinn and others 2000), while those across the border in Rwanda had an infection rate of less than 3 percent when they were jointly tested, is suggestive of a large benefit to couples testing.[14] Similarly, in two studies of discordant couples in Zambia, the couples without joint testing had a rate of infection of 20 percent (Hira and others 1990), compared to a rate of 7 percent among the couples with joint testing (Fideli and others 2001). Furthermore, the rate of infection among couples who are jointly tested and are both HIV negative was less than 1 percent in one study (Roth and others 2001).

One of the most frequently expressed fears about couples testing is that when the woman is positive, she will be stigmatized and abused. But in Zambia, fewer than 4 percent of discordant couples separated in the year after joint testing and counseling, a percentage that might be as low as the rate of separation in the absence of couples testing (Kempf and others 2008).

While studies have found counseling to be effective for couples in which one is HIV infected (Allen, Serufilira, Bogaerts, and others 1992; Allen, Tice, and others 1992; Allen, Serufilira, Gruber, and others 1993; Padian and others 1993; Roth and others 2001), it has an even more promising role for couples in which neither person is yet infected. Furthermore, a few studies suggest that people are more likely to accept couples counseling in their home than at health care facilities (Matovu and others 2002; Were and others 2003; Farquhar and others 2004). When couples learn each other's HIV status as well as their own and receive counseling about the dangers of unprotected sex outside the couple, such knowledge not only might increase condom use with other partners, but also might reduce the frequency of such partners. Thus, couples counseling, especially in the couple's home, might discourage the practice of multiple concurrent partnerships, which is thought to be a major contributor to the epidemic (Morris and Kretzschmar 1997; Halperin and Epstein 2004; Epstein 2007).

When comparing data from these various observational studies, the jointly tested couples are not necessarily comparable to the couples not jointly tested. The most prominent reason is that couples who accept joint testing and counseling may be exactly the ones who are most predisposed to safe behavior. But until a more rigorous evaluation shows otherwise, the established theory of asymmetric information and the observational evidence support a donor policy that favors couples testing over individual testing—and they strongly support the performance of more rigorous research on couples testing.

A country with the resources and the motivation to push HIV-prevention efforts beyond those at highest risk can expand door-to-door couples counseling by offering rewards to counselors based on the number of households reached and measures of the quality of counseling interventions. With appropriate quality controls and social audits, AIDS control programs can sub-contract couples counseling to NGOs, with rewards based on both quantity and quality of population coverage. These techniques have been used successfully in the cases of agricultural extension and house-to-house residual spraying for malaria.

Incentives to Use AIDS Treatment as HIV Prevention

Because effective AIDS treatment reduces the amount of HIV in the blood stream to undetectable levels, it has long been argued that AIDS treatment might itself constitute an effective HIV-prevention tool. Recently a group of authors based at the World Health Organization (WHO) published an article proposing a new "test-and-treat" policy in which every adult in a population is tested for HIV/AIDS and all who test positive immediately begin treatment, regardless of their CD4 count (Granich and others 2009). The authors argue that this approach can reverse the epidemic—and at lower cost than would universal treatment initiated years later relative to each patient's disease progression, at conventional CD4 thresholds. They base this conclusion on mathematical modeling using strong assumptions regarding the patients' adherence to medication for decades, despite having never been sick; the degree to which infectiousness is suppressed by ART; and a hypothetical reduction in risk behavior in the entire population that would accompany widespread treatment.

How much would the test-and-treat approach cost? As expected, it would be very expensive to implement. One way to show this is by juxtaposing test-and-treat scenarios to other ART scenarios in sub-Saharan Africa (figure 2-2). I distinguish scenarios by the treatment eligibility criterion, which is the number of CD4 cells per microliter of blood at which people are eligible for treatment, and by the proportion meeting that criterion who are added to treatment rolls in any year, which I call the "uptake rate." As further discussed in Chapter 3, from 2003 to 2006 when the eligibility criterion was 200 CD4 cells per microliter of blood, the average uptake rate in sub-Saharan Africa increased from about 15 to about 30 percent. To compute a lower estimate of the future costs to donors and governments, the first scenario explores an uptake rate of only 15 percent

FIGURE 2-2. Cost of Antiretroviral Therapy Options in Sub-Saharan Africa, 2010–50

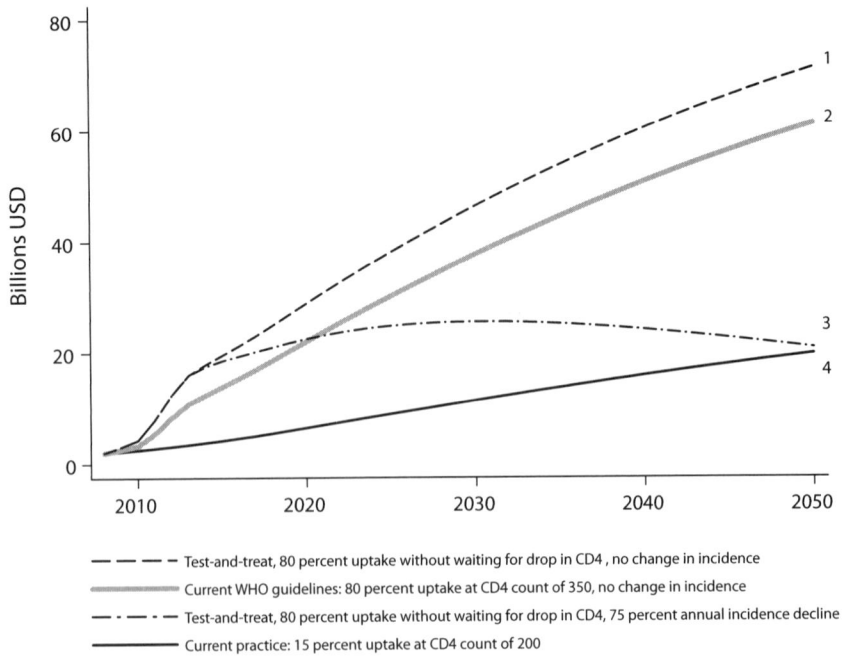

— — — — Test-and-treat, 80 percent uptake without waiting for drop in CD4 , no change in incidence

Current WHO guidelines: 80 percent uptake at CD4 count of 350, no change in incidence

— · — · — Test-and-treat, 80 percent uptake without waiting for drop in CD4, 75 percent annual incidence decline

Current practice: 15 percent uptake at CD4 count of 200

Source: Author's calculations.

of unmet need each future year, with the historical eligibility criterion of 200. As the bottom curve (number 4) in figure 2-2 shows, the cost of this ART policy would rise from about $4 billion in 2010 to almost $20 billion in 2050, with a present value of $211 billion through 2050 for AIDS treatment alone.

A second scenario illustrates what happens if governments follow the WHO's newly proposed CD4-count threshold of 350 cells per microliter and boost the uptake rate from the current 15 percent to 80 percent. As curve number 2 in figure 2-2 shows, assuming this more ambitious treatment regime is insufficient to reduce HIV incidence, the annual cost of expanding AIDS treatment would soar to $20 billion by 2020, and the present value of the costs through 2050 would hit $683 billion.

Now let us cost out the test-and-treat scenarios. The top curve (number 1) in figure 2-2 presents the projected cost of treating 80 percent of all HIV-infected people as soon as they become infected, without waiting for their CD4 counts to drop to 350, under the pessimistic assumption that such a policy would not actually reduce the incidence of new infections as intended. Curve number 3 projects the cost of treating 80 percent of the HIV-infected population, again without waiting for their CD4 counts to drop to 350, under the optimistic assumption that with this much coverage, the rate of new infections would decline precipitously by 75 percent per year. In this case, Africa would have no new infections after the year 2020. These two curves together establish upper and lower bounds on the possible future costs of the test-and-treat policy option, with the true future costs lying somewhere in between.

At least in the first decade of its implementation, the test-and-treat scenario would be even more expensive than a policy of 80 percent coverage at the WHO's new guidelines. Under either the optimistic or the pessimistic version of the test-and-treat option, annual treatment costs rise to $20 billion in the middle of the next decade, and aggregate discounted costs over the next forty years rise to between $536 billion and $849 billion. Thus, the test-and-treat option is between two-and-a-half and four times more expensive than continued expansion at the lower uptake rate and the lower eligibility criterion would be.

Moreover, the test-and-treat approach may fail in expensive ways. For example, recent meta-analysis has found that for people on ART, the number of infections per thousand person-years is about five, not very different from the infectivity of people not on ART during the decade or so beginning six to ten weeks after infection until the year before death (Attia and others 2009). Infections that do occur under test-and-treat would transmit a drug-resistant form of HIV that will be more expensive to treat than existing viruses. While most resistant viruses are less fit than "wild" or "naïve" HIV that has not been exposed to ART, the wide-scale implementation of the test-and-treat policy creates the opportunity for the virus to attempt trillions of additional experiments with alternative strategies for resistance, and it is plausible that one or more could lead to a resistant HIV that will be more virulent than the HIV-1 virus that currently infects more than 33 million people worldwide (Dodd, Garnett, and Hallett 2010).[15]

Although this analysis leads to skepticism about the feasibility and affordability of the test-and-treat policy option as a contributor to an AIDS transition, PBIs that strengthen AIDS treatment may contribute to slowing HIV transmission in more modest ways. For example, in the 5–10 percent of sub-Saharan African cohabiting partnerships with only one HIV-infected partner (Beegle and de Walque, 2009), PBIs to encourage early ART initiation and persistent ART adherence could overcome the infected partner's possible reluctance to taking medication when that person has never experienced symptoms, thereby preventing or postponing the spouse's infection.

Incentives to Mobilize AIDS Patients for HIV Prevention

The test-and-treat strategy discussed in the preceding section depends primarily on a biological effect of treatment to reduce the infectivity of the treated individual, but the original proponents of that strategy also hypothesized that universal treatment would somehow reduce the risk behavior not only of those on treatment but also of the general population. The alternative hypothesis is that easy and inexpensive access to treatment would reduce the risk of AIDS and thus "disinhibit" risk behavior (Over and others 2006). A study of ART patients in Côte d'Ivoire who were counseled to maintain safe behavior showed no increase in self-reported risk behavior (Katzenstein, Laga, and Moatti 2003). And a recent study in Rwanda finds the same encouraging result for patients using more reliable biological markers for unprotected sex (Dunkle and others 2008).

However, few studies have examined the more important impact of expanded treatment access on risk behavior of the much larger population of adults not yet on treatment or not even infected (Garnett and others 2010). A recent study of survey data from Mozambique found evidence that men's demand for risky sexual behaviors increases with the false belief that AIDS can be cured while women's increases with the correct belief that AIDS can be treated (de Walque, Kazianga, and Over 2010).

Instead of just hoping that expanded treatment access will promote safe sexual behavior in the broader community, the AIDS community can design programs to mobilize these patients—who are in good health because of their precise adherence to their medication regime—to become a vital channel for reaching out to the much larger population of people whose risk behavior places them in danger of infection. With proper training, motivation, and monitoring, patients can work to ensure that AIDS treatment does not engender complacency and disinhibition among non-patients but instead encourages reductions in risk behavior.

One way to leverage such patients into enhanced HIV prevention in the community is to apply PBIs to adherence support organizations, rather than to individual patients. An adherence support organization can be defined as an NGO that is dedicated to the objective of improving and sustaining treatment adherence of a defined group of patients, such as those receiving treatment from a given facility.[16] Along with their family members, the patients are often members of the organization. When multiple adherence support organizations exist in a community, their relative performance can be judged not only by their success at maintaining their members' adherence but also by their efforts to reach out to non-members with HIV-prevention interventions. A PBI reward structure can be constructed to reward both of these activities. The portion of an organization's funds that goes toward continuing support of its existing patients would be conditional only on the survival and continued membership of those patients. However, when new funding is needed to support newly recruited ART patients, the funder can allocate it to the adherence support organization that has recently demonstrated the most success in its prevention outreach to the surrounding community. Since the need for treatment is likely to be greatest near places where HIV transmission is most frequent, such as hot spots of risky sexual behavior or intravenous drug use, such a process of muted competition among adherence support organizations would leverage prevention efforts in the places that most need enhanced prevention as well as sustained treatment adherence.

Major Donors Do Not Use PBIs

A recent review of the PBIs currently deployed by the three major AIDS donors compares publicly available information on their use of such incentives (Oomman, Wendt, and Droggitis 2010). As that study shows, while all the donors express concern about performance, none publishes quantitative performance measures specific to the many HIV-prevention programs it supports that would make it possible to judge the contractor's achievement of HIV-prevention objectives. And none explicitly sets quantitative targets and then rewards individual implementers for achievement by a pre-agreed formula. Since at the aggregate level the most concrete indicator is the number of individuals receiving ART, all three donors implicitly bias their reporting against HIV prevention relative to treatment, and none explicitly addresses the problem of insufficient leadership for HIV prevention at the top levels of government.

PBIs are effective tools that good managers can use to improve the day-to-day performance of their staff or the compliance or adherence of their patients. However, PBIs alone are unlikely to be sufficient to generate the increased effort needed for an AIDS transition because these incentives do not typically address the constraints under which providers and their managers operate. Managers of health facilities may be unable to serve more patients because of interruptions in their supply chains. Or the managers of the supply chain, if offered a PBI for improved logistical support to health facilities, may be unable to respond because of problems with the national customs agency or lack of functional roads during the rainy season. Furthermore, even at the level of the provider–patient encounter, sometimes the reasons for poor results lie outside the control of individual providers or their managers. The provider's superiors may lack the authority, skills, resources, or motivation to review the provider's performance. Or the superiors may be frustrated by a lack of coordination from other parts of government. In these situations, improved and sustained motivation is needed at a higher level.

Counting the Saved: A "Cash-on-Delivery" Approach to HIV/AIDS Assistance

To succeed in holding down AIDS mortality for a decade or two while bringing new infections even lower, many communities, provinces, and nations will need to generate and maintain sustained cooperation between the multiple active and passive participants in HIV-prevention and AIDS-treatment activities. HIV/AIDS champions will need resources to recruit allies or dissuade opponents among parts of the society with a less direct stake in combating the epidemic. Donors and governments will need a policy instrument that will attract and reward the attention of the most innovative national thinkers. They also will need a policy instrument that directly supports the measurement required to track progress in reducing new HIV infections. And political leaders might value a policy instrument that could give them a pretext for urging their broad constituencies toward HIV-prevention effort even if most citizens are already behaving responsibly.

This section describes a policy instrument called "cash-on-delivery" (COD) aid that we at the Center for Global Development believe fulfills all these criteria. The approach centers on a COD contract between a donor and recipient country or state that stipulates an agreed-upon payment as a reward or prize that the recipient wins because of its achievement of a challenging, worthwhile, internationally recognized social objective. By contracting to pay a cash reward to the top level of government of $100 for every HIV infection averted, for example, the COD policy instrument is a powerfully motivating performance-based incentive.

Since the earliest days of the effort to contain the AIDS epidemic, public health experts have stressed that leadership of HIV-prevention efforts must come from the top of a country's political and social structure (Tarantola and Mann 1995). In those countries where highly placed leaders, such as the president, have forcibly and unabashedly addressed the AIDS epidemic, HIV infection rates have frequently fallen. Examples include Thailand, Brazil, Mexico, and Uganda. Yet the leaders of many countries with severe epidemics have turned their backs on HIV/AIDS control efforts, preferring to use their prestige in support of other goals. In other countries, national leadership has been to no avail because state and local leaders have refused to follow. The COD approach aims to help donors facilitate longer-term commitments to enduring effort by allowing governmental champions of HIV/AIDS prevention to allocate a portion of any cash award to sustain cooperation, recruit allies, or to dissuade opponents.

While current HIV/AIDS programs are designed to employ and promote "planners" who implement top-down approaches to AIDS control, a cash-on-delivery approach calls forth the innovative "seekers" (Easterly 2006) who will search for ways to most effectively prevent new infections in exchange for a promised reward. As explained in more detail below, COD does not just include but actually requires reliable and trustworthy measurement of new infections. And it offers to national and local political leaders a useful justification for promoting HIV prevention beyond what a short-sighted or prudish constituency might otherwise prefer.

Attributes of a COD Approach

The idea of a cash-on-delivery approach to HIV/AIDS prevention follows a proposal by Center for Global Development president Nancy Birdsall and colleagues to apply cash incentives to foreign aid more broadly (Barder and Birdsall 2006; Birdsall and Savedoff 2010). For example, Birdsall and a coauthor suggest that a payment of $200 per child be made to the recipient government for every additional child above an agreed baseline who completes primary school and takes a test (Birdsall and Savedoff 2010, p. 55). To ensure host-country agreement with the COD contract, all donors should agree that these payments would be over and above the existing education assistance funding in the country, not a substitute for it. The COD contract requires that audited measures of the specified outcomes be made prior to the contract's start and then periodically to establish the gains to be rewarded.

COD differs from PBI approaches on the level and the time frame of the outcomes to be rewarded and on the degree of funders' involvement in the day-to-day production process. COD applies incentives to the top levels of governmental organization, such as the state, province, or nation. And it recognizes that the leaders of national and state governments in recipient countries must constantly balance the demands from a long list of constituencies and clients. Given dynamic and even chaotic political environments, agreements made years earlier to sustain an HIV-prevention effort easily may become less urgent than the concerns of the day.

Whereas PBIs reward relatively short-term, monthly, or quarterly improvements in patient-level or facility-level outcomes, the time frame of the COD approach is to reward medium-term, annual, or multiyear improvements in the average outcome for an entire state or national population. Because PBIs integrate with the day-to-day management of individual interventions, the donor typically becomes involved in selecting the inputs, outputs, or activities to be monitored and rewarded. In contrast, the COD approach is removed from the process and agnostic regarding the contribution to the outcome of individual interventions.

The promise that an economic incentive offered to an entire population might induce individuals to participate in a successful disease-prevention program is suggested by the true story of an island in the South Pacific that eliminated malaria in the 1990s. The inhabitants of Aneityum, an island of the nation of Vanuatu, traditionally tolerated endemic malaria, with its periodic bouts of fever and occasional childhood deaths. In the 1980s, their island lifestyle was enriched by biannual visits of a cruise ship and its free-spending tourists. Then in 1990, two tourists contracted malaria. While it was unclear whether the passengers were infected during the visit to Aneityum or another island, the cruise-ship captain refused to return until the island was malaria free.[17] Journal articles document how the extraordinary community-level motivation and participation of the Aneityum population led to the successful elimination of malaria on the island (Atkinson and others 2010; Kaneko and others 2000; and Kaneko 2010).

Although malaria is different from HIV in many respects, misalignment of individual and social incentives contributes to the spread of both diseases. For many people, the private benefits of preventive behavior are insufficient compared to the immediate discomfort, cost, or inconvenience they entail. Furthermore, effective prevention of both diseases requires the coordination of many government and non-government agents throughout society. If the promise of cruise-ship spending could change the balance of incentives in favor of controlling malaria, perhaps a COD approach could work a similar miracle for HIV prevention.

The COD approach has been developed and proposed for application in other sectors in response to four intellectual currents that are common to the field of foreign assistance in general and to HIV prevention in particular. The first is a trend toward results-based foreign assistance, exemplified by the U.S. government's Millennium Challenge Corporation (Radelet 2003), the Global Alliance for Vaccines and Immunization, and the PBI movement (Eichler, Levine, and Performance-Based Incentives Working Group 2009). Second is a growing belief among some observers that in the field of development, the foreign "planners" have less pertinent knowledge and are less important for success than the local "seekers," as described above (Easterly 2006). Third, an increasing number of observers have wondered whether the poor results achieved by public-service delivery in low-income countries can be attributed partly to insufficient motivation at higher as well as lower levels of public-service delivery institutions (Filmer and Pritchett 1999). Fourth, in the domain of HIV prevention, data on the cost of service delivery reveal enormous unexplained variation in unit costs for the delivery of the same service within and across countries, suggesting substantial scope for enhanced incentives to improve the prevention results obtained from available prevention resources (Marseille and others 2004, 2007; Dandona, Sisodia, Kumar, and others 2005; Dandona, Sisodia, Prasad, and others 2005; Dandona, Ramesh, and others 2005; Guinness and others 2005; Bautista-Arredondo and others 2008).

How would COD payments work? There are five key features, as box 2-3 shows. The first is that a donor (bilateral, multilateral, or philanthropic) and recipient (national or state government) enter into an agreement in which the donor agrees to reward the recipient country if it achieves, or proportional to its achievement of, a certain development outcome. In development-speak, "outcomes" are a fundamental dimension of peoples' well-being, such as poverty reduction, nutritional status, cognitive development, educational achievement, and health status. Thus, as distinct from financing budget support, inputs, or activities, the COD approach pays only for evidence that development itself has been advanced.

The COD payment would not substitute for traditional input-based foreign assistance. Nor would the payment be conditional on any government policy decisions, enacted legislation, or implemented regulation. For example, suppose an HIV-prevention effort involves the ministries of health, education, and civil society. A typical National AIDS Control Program would include a detailed list of activities that each ministry would perform ("outputs") and would budget the vehicles, materials, training, and logistical support ("inputs") thought necessary to produce these outputs. Such a plan might mention a reduction in new HIV infections as an aspiration or even an objective. But the ministries in charge of executing the plan would only be held accountable for the specified inputs and outputs.

In contrast, the COD approach eschews any detailed programming of the outputs or activities of the individual government agencies. It does not seek to hold the separate agencies accountable for their activities or outputs, nor does it seek to attribute any changes in the outcome to any individual or institutional actors. It also would not specify how any prize would be distributed among the local actors who have contributed to winning it. A recipient government might best leverage a COD agreement into HIV-prevention achievements by openly discussing the prize distribution

---

BOX 2-3. A Snapshot of the Cash-on-Delivery Approach

Key Features

Rewards improvements in fundamental dimensions of human well-being ("outcomes")

Takes a hands-off approach to administration: donor does not prescribe how outcomes are to be achieved

Independently verifies outcomes

Is transparent

Complements other aid programs

Basic Steps

Two parties negotiate and sign a medium-term contract specifying output-performance goals

Recipient government collects and reports output data using mutually agreed sampling methods[1]

Donor independently audits measured output

Donor pays recipient according to achievement of previously negotiated output-performance goals

Operational or impact evaluation research is optional, potentially funded by a third party

---

Source: Author's adaptation of Birdsall and Savedoff 2010, figure 3.
1. The agreement must specify at least the population to be sampled, the sampling frame, the clustering method, the sample size and distribution across clusters, and the timing of the baseline and of successive follow-up surveys.

---

with constituent local governments and civil society groups—which would encourage buy-in at the community level. Depending on the recipient's perception of where incentives would do the most good, the recipient might offer to distribute portions of the prize to local government health officials, NGOs, mayors, or even individual citizens.

The other four features include "hands-off" administration of the program, independent verification of outcomes, transparency, and complementarity with other aid programs. In this context, "hands-off" means that the COD agreement would not necessarily provide technical assistance, advice, training, oversight, or any other input to program execution. Host-country governments and their existing advisors would be free to seek any of the inputs they deem useful to obtaining the contractually agreed improvements, but no additional budget would be available from the COD process for this assistance. And most important, the recipient government would not be required to spend COD payments from the donor on the program, or even the sector, on which the payments are conditioned. As a result, the government could use the extra resources from a COD program on HIV prevention to build roads, improve sanitation, or even train its national soccer team.

The COD approach also involves five basic steps, outlined in box 2-3. That the fifth step—operational or impact evaluation research—is optional clearly distinguishes the COD performance audits from formal impact evaluation. While the objective of impact evaluation is to determine whether a specific intervention has improved a development outcome relative to a "counterfactual" state of the world in which that intervention was not implemented, the more modest objective of the COD approach is to simply determine whether improvement has occurred relative to a benchmark and, if so, to estimate the magnitude of the improvement.

By comparing the future value of a development outcome to a benchmark and agreeing to pay for every unit by which the outcome is better than the benchmark, the COD approach provides an incentive to exert effort toward improving the outcome regardless of whether the selected benchmark accurately represents the counterfactual. The COD approach is thus useful in contexts where impact evaluation would be infeasible either politically or technically. For example, impact evaluation is notoriously handicapped when a development outcome is affected by many contextual variables, only some of which are under the control of the evaluators and some of which cannot even be measured (Deaton 2009). The COD program has no such handicap because it rewards governments based on outcome improvements, whatever the cause of those improvements. Impact evaluation typically requires that interventions be applied to a random sample of subjects or communities and withheld from a matched comparator group that does not receive the intervention. The COD approach requires only that the index whose improvement is to be rewarded be measured at least twice, once at the baseline to establish a benchmark and once in a follow-up survey.

Although the COD approach eschews a research perspective, it may indirectly encourage research.[18] To the extent that the COD approach motivates the recipient government to learn what works best to achieve the COD-determined improvement objectives, the government and its partners are free to conduct research to that end. Indeed, because it is motivated to improve the COD outcomes, the government may pay new attention to relevant existing research and show new interest in eliciting relevant operational research from the academic community.

COD for HIV Prevention

So how would we design a COD contract for HIV prevention?[19] Such an approach holds great promise but also faces serious challenges. First, the subject population for HIV prevention is potentially quite large, consisting of everyone whose behavior places him or her at risk of infection or of infecting someone else. As a result, a COD contract will have to pay the rewards based on a sample of the relevant population rather than on the kind of comprehensive administrative data that could be used in a COD for education—or even for an AIDS treatment program (which would have a relatively smaller cohort).

Second, while the donor is paying to avert an HIV infection, it is a relatively rare event compared to, for example, failure to complete primary school. Whereas the risk of HIV infection in a general population is typically less than 1 percent per year and almost never more than 2 percent per year, as many as one-third of children in a low-income country may fail to complete primary school (Birdsall and Savedoff 2010). While rarity of new infections is the intended goal, the challenge is that the rarer the event is, the larger is the sample size needed to detect a reduction in its frequency. A larger sample size costs more and allows for the possibility of mistakes—or even opportunistic manipulation of the measurements.

Third, defining precisely what constitutes a commendable outcome is difficult in the case of HIV. In Birdsall and Savedoff's example of a COD contract to improve education, primary school completion is a successful result, worthy of reward for its own sake. However, in the case of HIV infection, donors want to commend and reward the recipient for averting HIV infections. HIV infections averted can be defined only in reference to a counterfactual state of the world in which they would have occurred. Specifically, the number of HIV infections averted is defined as the arithmetic difference between the number of new HIV infections that have occurred over a certain period of time in a certain population and the number that would have occurred in the same period and the same population, but in the counterfactual state of the world.

The COD approach is to reward any improvement—in this case, any reduction in new infections—beyond some specified threshold without regard to why that improvement occurred or whether it would have occurred in the absence of the COD program. This could be characterized as the adoption of a naïve counterfactual that no change would have occurred without the COD program or simply as the recognition that the donor values the improvement for its own sake and is willing to reward the country for the achievement whatever the cause. Adopting this approach for an infectious disease is complicated by the fact that for any infectious disease, the incidence rate—that is, the fraction of an uninfected population that becomes infected over a given interval—varies substantially over time even in the absence of intervention. As depicted in figure 1-1 at the beginning of this book, the incidence of new infections is typically high in the early stages of the epidemic when the entire population is susceptible. It then declines as the prevalence rate of the disease rises and the formerly susceptible population is saturated with infection. The incidence rate then can increase again as new cohorts of susceptible people enter the population. The time scale of these cycles varies from weeks for influenza to years for HIV.

The advent of effective, accessible ART for AIDS patients adds another difficulty to the interpretation of trends in the prevalence rate because an increase in prevalence could be caused either by prevention failure or by treatment success. It would be logically contradictory to reward a country for extending the lives of AIDS patients—as we propose in the next chapter to do with a COD program for AIDS treatment—while simultaneously rewarding it for reducing the proportion of its population living with HIV/AIDS in the name of HIV prevention.

Because of these complications, using the COD approach for HIV prevention requires more attention to defining the benchmark than would be the case when applying the COD approach to other development outcomes, including access to AIDS treatment. This third characteristic of HIV prevention is the most challenging impediment to operating a COD program for HIV prevention. But it, too, is surmountable if the donor and recipient can agree at the outset on the use of the statistical, modeling, and auditing methods that will enable the donor to pay a reward commensurate with the recipient's real achievements in HIV prevention.

Defining a plausible counterfactual against which to measure the number of averted HIV infections has two feasible approaches: the prevalence modeling approach and the test-of-recent-infection (TRI) approach.

THE PREVALENCE MODELING APPROACH. The first approach involves combining a detailed model of the epidemic with measurements of the prevalence rate in two surveys of the general population—one before the intervention begins and the other after the agreed time for the intervention has lapsed. Supplementing this information are prevalence data from earlier years, convenience samples at antenatal clinics, and data on the number receiving ART. Together, these data are used to infer the actual rate of new infections in the interval and the rate of new infections that would have occurred in the absence of behavioral change. The difference between these two rates as a proportion of the population provides an estimate of the number of HIV infections averted.

As an example, suppose that in a hypothetical country with a high HIV prevalence rate, surveillance has been conducted at nine antenatal clinics since 1989, and a baseline survey of HIV infection in 8,000 households was conducted in 2002 (Hallett, Gregson, and others 2009). Based on these data and expert opinion regarding the earlier history of the epidemic, a model would predict a stabilization or a slight reduction in HIV prevalence in the absence of any change in risk behavior or increase in AIDS treatment, owing to the natural evolution of an epidemic of infectious disease as the most susceptible people in the population become infected, and some die. This prediction becomes the counterfactual against which the country's prevention performance will be measured.

Now suppose that the country signs a COD contract with a donor in 2002, in which the donor agrees to reward the recipient country $10 for every HIV infection averted by 2007. Subsequent surveillance of the nine clinics and estimates from a 2007 follow-up household survey would provide the data to be measured against the counterfactual. Combining the 2007 data with known rates of AIDS treatment gives an estimation of the number of HIV infections that may have been averted because of changes in risk behavior. If the country achieves a probable reduction in HIV prevalence much greater than would be expected with no change—say between 140,000 and 270,000 averted HIV infections, with a best estimate of 210,000—the donor would pay for that improved performance—in this case $2.1 million.

The question arises whether the payout should be diminished because of the large uncertainty around this estimate of averted infections. To the degree that the uncertainty is a result of the donor's unwillingness to finance larger samples for the household surveys, the recipient government should not be held accountable for the lack of precision. But in this example, the fact that the prevalence rates vary from one antenatal clinic to another increases uncertainty. To reward countries for greater precision in the follow-up prevalence estimate, the payout rule could be revised to deduct for imprecision. For example, the original agreement could be to pay $15 per infection averted less $5 per infection for the difference between the upper and lower limits on the 95 percent confidence limits. In this example, the recipient government would receive $3.15 million less $650,000 for a net payment of $2.5 million.

The prevalence modeling approach has the advantage of feasibility with existing HIV testing and survey methods but has several disadvantages. The main drawback is the complexity of the process needed to construct and use a counterfactual to interpret trends in prevalence. Modelers can adjust the mathematical modeling method to be conservative by raising the threshold for finding evidence of behavior change that affects the course of the epidemic, or they can adjust the model to be more generous. This flexibility opens the calculation of HIV infections to dispute. Another disadvantage is the strong influence on the estimates of HIV infections averted of early HIV infection data collected before a surveillance system was established. This makes the analysis vulnerable to gaming. In addition, the increasing availability of ART that sustains HIV prevalence in the population requires additional complex adjustments to the prevalence modeling.[20]

The original COD agreement could address these disadvantages by establishing an objective expert panel to which the donor and the recipient would defer and a binding arbitration mechanism in case of subsequent disagreements. And even with these vulnerabilities, the prevalence modeling approach might be less subject to opportunism than current, input-based, aid modalities. Indeed, the establishment of such mechanisms might be advisable for any COD agreement. Nevertheless, an alternative approach that depends less on modeling and more on direct measurement would be desirable.

THE "TEST-OF-RECENT-INFECTIONS" APPROACH. The second approach makes use of blood tests that detect whether an HIV-infected person has become infected within a specific recent period of time, such as six months. After a decade of research, these tests of recent infection are on the verge of gaining approval for wider use. By using such a test to measure HIV incidence directly instead of inferring it from a change in prevalence, a COD program for HIV prevention can conform more closely to the COD norm by simply paying for any difference in directly measured recent infections between a baseline and follow-up survey.

The original TRI method judges when an HIV-infected person was infected by applying a more and less sensitive test to the same blood specimen. On the theory that the reactivity of the test to the blood sample increases with the length of time the person has been infected, researchers use as a measure of those newly infected the number of people who scored HIV-positive on the more sensitive test but HIV-negative on the less sensitive one. A newer TRI method gauges the time since infection by measuring the opacity of a single blood specimen. While both methods show promise, they suffer from the same problem when used alone: some people who have been infected a long time appear on the test to be recently infected, thus biasing upward the measured rate of HIV incidence.[21] Furthermore, the proportion of such people turns out to vary from one epidemiologic setting to another. Recently researchers have shown that these problems can be addressed by using several tests on the same blood sample.[22] As a result of this more accurate combination testing, donors can use TRI to reward countries for reducing HIV incidence.

By delinking rewards for HIV prevention from prevalence measurement, the TRI approach shields COD for HIV prevention from the charge that it could discourage countries from prolonging the lives of people living with HIV/AIDS. Because it is direct, the TRI approach reduces the dependence of any COD payout rule on complex epidemiologic modeling.[23] While application of the TRI approach might occasionally lead the donor to pay a recipient for incidence reductions that are part of the natural epidemic cycle, this problem is generic to the COD approach and can be addressed through the appropriate design of the payout rule.

The one problem that the TRI approach aggravates in comparison to prevalence modeling is the difficult requirement for a large sample or a long period between the baseline and follow-up surveys. In the prevalence modeling example discussed above, when prevalence has declined by 20 percent, two samples of 8,000 each at a five-year interval are sufficient to reject the hypothesis that prevalence is unchanged on 80 percent of repetitions.[24] However, with the TRI approach, because the incidence rate is much smaller than the prevalence rate, either the sample size or the number of years between surveys must be larger to detect any given improvement.

The sample size and survey interval requirements for capturing an annual reduction in incidence depend on several factors that vary across countries and epidemiological contexts. Suppose the COD criterion is that a reward be paid if a second incidence survey yields an estimated incidence that is statistically smaller than the incidence in the baseline survey. In this situation, figure 2-3 depicts the trade-off between sample size and survey interval to allow a COD reward to be paid. The curved lines depict the level sets of equal statistical power with lines to the top-right indicating higher statistical power for rejecting the hypothesis of equal incidence as either sample size or the time between surveys gets larger.

When the starting incidence is relatively high at two new infections per hundred person-years and the actual decline is large at 40 percent per year, as depicted in panel d, a powerful test can be achieved with a relatively

FIGURE 2-3. Statistical Power as a Function of Survey Interval and Sample Size

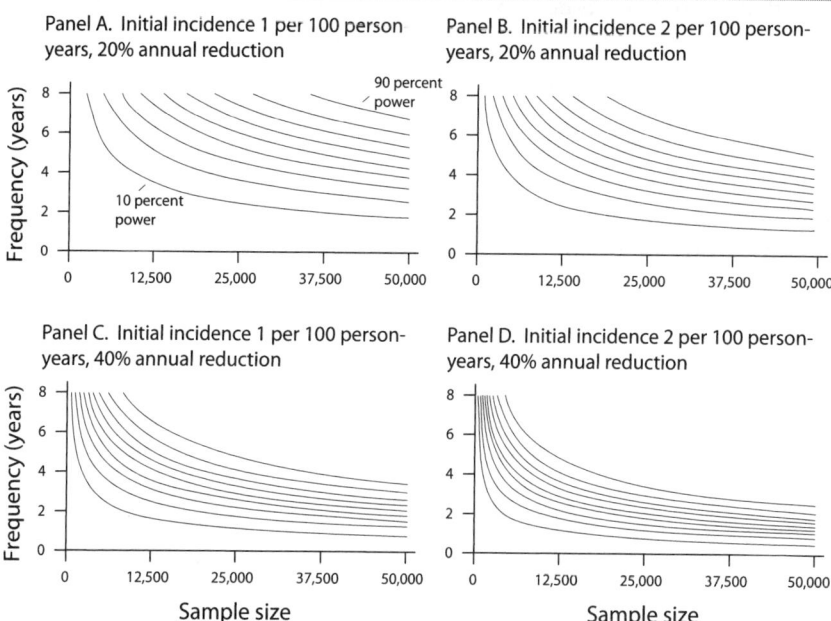

Panel A. Initial incidence 1 per 100 person years, 20% annual reduction

Panel B. Initial incidence 2 per 100 person-years, 20% annual reduction

Panel C. Initial incidence 1 per 100 person-years, 40% annual reduction

Panel D. Initial incidence 2 per 100 person-years, 40% annual reduction

Note: The curved lines depict statistical power, from 10 percent power to 90 percent.

Source: Hallett and Over (2010).

small sample of 25,000 individuals and a relatively short interval between surveys of four years.[25] But when the starting incidence is relatively low at only one new infection per hundred person-years and the true reduction is rather small at only 20 percent, as depicted in panel a, a relatively large sample of 50,000 and a relatively long interval between surveys of six years would be required to obtain the same statistical power. Of course, a larger sample and a longer interval would be more costly, but choosing a payout rule that increases the payout smoothly with increases in the estimated number of HIV infections averted would alleviate the cost to some extent. Thus, even if sampling error leads to an underestimate of the country's reduction in HIV incidence, the probability exists of some payout. Furthermore, a smoothly increasing payout rule will motivate the recipient country planners to reduce prevalence as much as they can.

Payout Rules

Regardless of the approach used to measure averted HIV infections, the payout can be a smoothly increasing function of the total number of HIV infections averted. In discussing the prevalence modeling approach, I suggest that payout could be $15 dollars for every averted infection, minus a $5 penalty for every unit difference between the high and low estimate boundaries of the 95 percent confidence interval.

Instead of a penalty for imprecision, the payout might include a bonus for precision. Figure 2-4 graphs the expected performance of four payout rules as a function of the true incidence reduction the recipient manages to achieve. The graph is constructed by averaging the payouts over many replications at each of a range of actual changes in the HIV incidence rate when the baseline and follow-up surveys include 20,000 subjects, the starting incidence is two new cases per 100 person-years (or 2 percent), and the interval between surveys is five years. The horizontal axis measures improvement, with the area right of zero representing up to a 50 percent reduction in incidence. The area left of zero represents a worsening of the situation, with a greater incidence of infection at the follow-up survey than at the baseline. The four curves represent the different payout rules, described below.

Since sample surveys by their nature do not count everyone, even a sample as large as 20,000 people can by chance be unrepresentative and yield an estimated decline in incidence when incidence has not truly declined. All the payout rules contain that possibility because the expected, or average, payouts are greater than zero even when the actual change in incidence is zero or positive. Including a COD agreement in the payout rule requires weighing the danger of overpayment against the danger of underpayment, which occurs when an unlucky sample underreports a country's true reduction of infection incidence. The possibility of over- or underpayment is inescapable in the context of a one-time COD program but becomes less important if the COD program is repeated with the same recipient.[26]

Payout rule 1 is a simple linear function of the incidence reduction that reaches its maximum when a country reduces incidence by half. The rationale for this maximum is that reducing incidence by half is a prodigious accomplishment for which donors would want to offer their maximum reward. But if the donor is willing to risk larger payouts, the threshold at which payout reaches its maximum could be adjusted to a 75 percent reduction or even a 100 percent reduction, without reducing the reward for a 50 percent reduction. Figure 2-4 shows that payout rule 1 risks only a small danger of overpayment (the region to the left of the zero) and then increases the recipient's expected reward in a roughly linear way up to the maximum of 50 percent.

Rule 2 differs from rule 1 only by offering the recipient a bonus for achieving a statistically significant reduction in incidence. Statistical signifi-

FIGURE 2-4. Relationship between Reductions in HIV Incidence and Expected Payout under Four Payout Rules

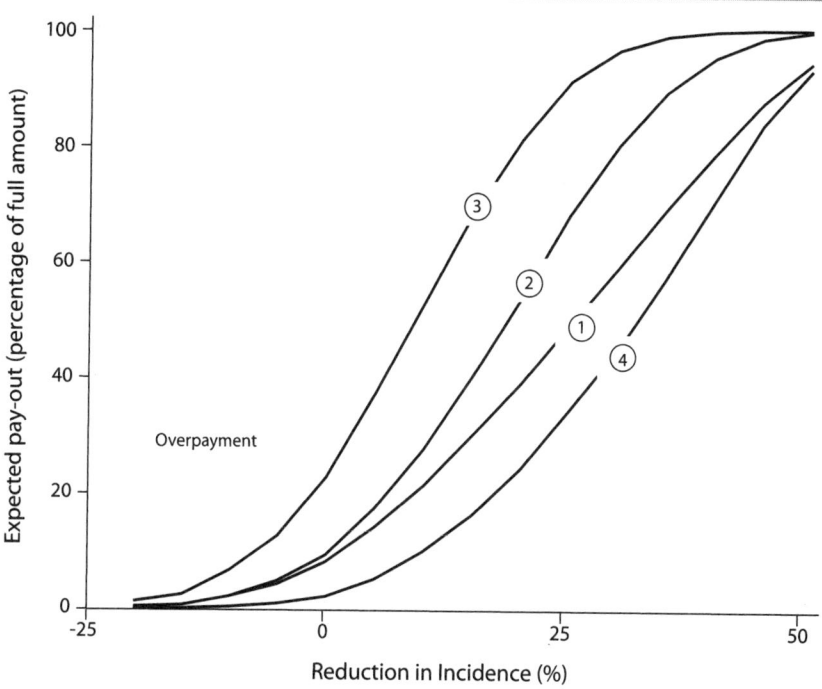

Rule 1: Pay out linearly in proportion to the reduction in incidence (up to a reduction by half)

Rule 2: Pay out linearly in proportion to the reduction in incidence (up to a reduction by half), with a bonus if the reduction reaches statistical significance at p=0.05

Rule 3: Pay out convexly (faster return at smaller reductions) in proportion to the reduction in incidence (up to a reduction by half), with a bonus if the reduction reaches statistical significance at p=0.05

Rule 4: Pay out concavely (faster increase in return at larger reductions) in proportion to the reduction in incidence (up to a reduction by half), with a bonus if the reduction reaches statistical significance at p=0.05.

Source: Hallett and Over (2010).

cance could be improved at any given level of incidence reduction by either increasing the sample size—a decision that the donor and recipient would make jointly and the donor presumably would fund—or improving the consistency of HIV prevention across the regions where incidence is measured. By reducing the variance in incidence reduction, the recipient government can improve the precision with which any given reduction is measured, thereby increasing the chance that it will win the precision bonus. Another way to improve the chance that the reduction will be statistically significant is for the reduction to be as large as possible, an additional incentive to the recipient to excel at HIV prevention. Figure 2-4 shows that the bonus makes the payout rule steeper until an inflection point at about a 20 percent reduction. Each incremental percentage point of reduction receives a greater reward under rule 2 than rule 1. With the same payment per estimated infection averted, the donor's expected cost is correspondingly greater.

Rule 3 is a modification of rule 2 designed to make the payout rule even steeper over the range of small improvements. This rule will be useful in encouraging performance in contexts where any reduction is extremely difficult. However, it provides an expected payout of 20 percent of the maximum when there has been no actual reduction in incidence. And more than rules 1 or 2, it risks payout when true incidence has increased.

Rule 4 demonstrates a payout rule that is less steep for small improvements and correspondingly steeper for large improvements. This rule could be useful when the donor and the recipient remain engaged in a succession of repeated COD programs for the same population. Perhaps in the early years, a very steep and forgiving payout rule like rule 3 would be best to motivate the recipient as it launches its enhanced HIV-prevention program. But then subsequent contracts could be more demanding, looking more like rule 2, 1, or even 4, to shift the steepest part of the payout rule to the more ambitious levels of incidence reduction.

Synergy between HIV Prevention and AIDS Treatment

A COD program for HIV prevention would be an even larger improvement over current donor practice than would be true for a COD program in AIDS treatment—which is elaborated in chapter 3 on treatment. Typical prevention programs measure only their inputs, such as the number of condoms distributed or man-hours of outreach time. They began reporting even the crudest measures of their coverage to the UN General Assembly for the first time in 2008. The COD approach would break new ground in rewarding prevention outcomes and providing HIV-prevention program managers with recent data on HIV incidence, an indicator of prevention success. Furthermore, the still-contentious debate over the relative benefits of different mixes of prevention programs in a "combination prevention package" would pass from the donor's responsibility to that of the recipient government. COD also would reward "seekers" rather than "planners" (Easterly 2006).

That said, there is enormous scope for taking advantage of the synergy between HIV prevention and AIDS treatment. HIV prevention costs money and effort today but only saves money on AIDS treatment years in the future, when the person whose infection has been averted would otherwise have become ill. This fact biases myopic governments away from effective HIV prevention. The weight assigned to prevention in the COD reward function will be subject to negotiation between donors and a given country recipient and may vary from country to country. But any positive weight given to prevention offers the recipient country a chance to reap immediate financial rewards for prevention accomplishments instead of having to wait for that reward until the infected person would have become sick.

The COD approach has the additional advantage over programmatic funding of giving the recipient country the incentive to seek out ways to increase the synergy between prevention and treatment. After all, if the country can more effectively leverage treatment efforts to motivate prevention, it increases its reward without having to spend more on prevention. Or if investing in improved roads has knock-on benefits on both prevention and treatment, again the country wins.

Once a group of donors has negotiated a COD contract covering both treatment and prevention—the two targets of an AIDS transition—all parties might agree to allow excluded donors to buy into the arrangement by adding to the unit payout for prevention or treatment. These additional donors effectively would bid upward the price or reward for prevention, treatment, or both. This kind of simulated market would reveal donors' preferences between these two interventions while adding to the recipient's incentive to do both.[27]

Potential Vulnerabilities of COD for AIDS Prevention and Their Remedies

The COD approach to HIV prevention has four potential weaknesses that must be addressed and remedied in any application. All existing forms of foreign assistance in general, and HIV/AIDS assistance policies in particular, share these vulnerabilities.

NEGOTIATION COSTS. COD requires that donors and recipients agree in advance on a precisely defined reward structure or payout function. In most countries, nongovernmental stakeholders also must be involved in this process to increase the chance that some rewards from the payout rule will pass through the government to those who are implementing the program. Their involvement also is necessary to ensure that those stakeholders with the most to contribute to HIV prevention can negotiate their share of the COD reward. The recipient government is likely to be most successful in maximizing its COD receipts if it uses the prospective receipts to achieve buy-in from these stakeholders. Negotiating these agreements will thus be a costly process, but perhaps no more so than in the case of conventional assistance programs. Given the prospect of these domestic transaction costs, the government that accepts a donor's offer to negotiate a COD agreement will likely be one whose leaders are strongly motivated to reduce HIV incidence and view the sharing of COD rewards with other stakeholders as a useful inducement to their energetic participation toward the common HIV prevention goal. Other governments need not apply.

MEASUREMENT OF OUTCOMES. The COD approach is not able to reward unmeasured improvements in population well-being and is thus biased against such unmeasured outcomes. Yet by using either of the proposed approaches to measure recent HIV infections and disclosing that information to the public, the recipient government inadvertently can stigmatize those practicing risky sexual behaviors. A recent flurry of reports that governments are persecuting men who have sex with men in African countries give credence to the possibility that each new cohort of government parliamentarians and policymakers is susceptible to the misconception that AIDS can be controlled by punishing those with high-risk behavior (Tarantola and others 2006).

As a result, to a greater degree than with other COD applications—such as improving school completion or reducing infant mortality—donors and recipients will need to agree to monitor HIV-prevention activities for human rights abuses.[28] If a donor is concerned that a country entering into a contract designed to reward a reduction in the number of new infections might carry out prevention programs that would infringe the human rights of its population, it can impose eligibility requirements, such as human-rights ombudsmen or civil-society watchdogs. Furthermore, donors can include in the contract a provision that overtly discriminatory or stigmatizing behavior toward the HIV-infected or the most at-risk populations, certified by a designated third party, will reduce or the COD payment.

Another tactic is to keep the size of the reward small in relation to the domestically borne costs of the prevention activities that the recipient is most likely to undertake and to the largest other conventionally financed flows into the country. The trick will be to choose a magnitude that is large enough to motivate people who attach intrinsic value to achieving the designated goal but not so large that it can attract the rent-seekers from other, more remunerative targets or elicit stigmatizing reactions toward those perceived as transmission risks.

BIG-COUNTRY BIAS. To the extent that improved implementation of treatment and prevention programs requires learning what works in each country, a big country might be better at improving. Natural variation of the program over its larger number of districts produces more extremes of performance in both directions. A large country has more skilled operations research personnel to investigate these good and bad performers and help disseminate lessons from the good ones. And big countries generally have more incentive to invest in knowledge because they have larger populations to reap these public good benefits. Parallel investments in small-country capacity can compensate for these biases and perhaps so can rewarding small countries even more for every unit improvement in either the treatment or the prevention dimension.

DISHONEST DATA COLLECTION AND ANALYSIS. The parties to a COD contract must agree on an arrangement to measure the key outcomes that will determine the payment. Because all COD contracts will reward achievement, they will create incentives for biased data collection and analysis. After the exacerbation of human rights abuses, one of the worst possible unintended consequences of implementing COD would be the corruption of the national statistics institutions. The exercise of due diligence to ensure that the COD outcomes are honestly measured is the most important responsibility of those designing the COD contract.

Several safeguards should be built in to protect the integrity of the COD outcome measurement process. The COD contract can include the provision that accredited international statistics organizations, either exclusively or in partnership with external agencies and local partners, perform surveys, data collection, and analysis. Household surveys can collect data not only on HIV incidence but also on individual characteristics and program variables, such as the local presence of HIV-prevention activities. These surveys can be used to guard against cheating in two ways. First, statisticians can confirm that the baseline and the follow-up samples contain similar distributions by age, sex, geographical location, and profession to be sure that any measured changes in incidence are not simply owing to a biased selection of one sample. Second, statisticians can confirm that correlations among the individual and program variables on the first survey are either unchanged in the second survey or are changed in plausible ways that an auditor who revisits a few of the sampled villages can confirm.

The security of blood samples should be guarded with particular care, and spot verification with DNA testing can be used to ensure that each blood sample is unique. In addition, the survey data can include codes to individually identify which survey employees administered, supervised, and keypunched each individual survey. In the history of household surveys, this last precaution has proved important in uncovering survey anomalies that have been introduced by sloth, incompetence, or corruption.[29]

Building in the proper safeguards at the time of COD contract negotiation may seem onerous, unnecessary, and even embarrassing. But the prospect of unintended consequences from the COD agreement—or even of the suspicion that COD outcome measurement has been suborned—should be sufficient to convince all parties of the need for these legalistic procedures. The objective is to ensure that the COD program, and the HIV-prevention programs it will reward, repel those individuals in any society with a predilection to falsifying data to achieve an illusory success. Instead, it will attract and ultimately reward those people in that same society who are most competent at, and passionately committed to, strengthening AIDS treatment and averting HIV infections.

Piloting a COD AIDS-Prevention Assistance Program

If the idea of using a COD reward for HIV-incidence reduction catches the imagination of one or more donors—and if countries where many of the HIV-prevention input and activity budgets are already financed are interested in reaching for this prize—there would be much to gain from piloting this idea in a country, or perhaps in a region of a country. A regional focus has the advantage of allowing comparisons with other regions that do not yet have a COD program. Unless the selection of regions to include in the pilot is entirely random, the comparison would have to match regions that receive the pilot to those that do not.

If a COD program is piloted in a region, those negotiating the COD contract should agree on a payout rule that rewards national and regional stakeholders. With some rewards going to national stakeholders, national decisionmakers will have more incentive to focus the best expertise available nationwide on the problem of improving results in the specific pilot region. Since measurement is likely to be challenging for any COD program, piloting in a region would enable the country and the donors to test the selected independent measurement agency to see if its performance is adequate and if it can remain immune to the temptation to exaggerate improvements. An important aspect of the pilot would be to test the feasibility and desirability of a specific reward or payout rule. After several years of successful implementation in pilot regions, the program could then be extended to the entire country.

Potential Fiscal Savings from Better Prevention

In the various countries of the world, the fiscal burden associated with lifetime AIDS treatment of an additional HIV-infected person, discounted at a social discount rate of 3 percent to the date of HIV infection, ranges from $5,000 in the poorest countries to more than $50,000 in the middle-income countries.[30] So preventing a person from becoming HIV infected during his or her lifetime is worth at least this much. If the world recognizes that each averted infection prevents that person from infecting others—and if it believes that an additional year of an adult's life averts orphanhood years, increases economic productivity, and lowers risk of social unrest—these dollar estimates are lower bounds for the value of averting an infection. Furthermore, a high rate of HIV infection casts an ominous shadow over the maturation of all the youth in the country, weakens the labor force, and worsens the investment climate by threatening potential foreign investors with high health care expenditures. Universal access to government-financed AIDS treatment, as is available in Botswana and Thailand, only partially mitigates this depressing effect. Effective HIV prevention, in contrast to universal treatment access, can prevent this disheartening future altogether.

Take the case of Thailand. During the 1990s, Thailand spent a total of about $434 million on its HIV program, most of which was on prevention (Over, Revenga, and others 2007; Revenga and others 2006). During this time period, HIV infection slowed substantially from its previous rate. By 2002, when Thailand introduced universal AIDS treatment, the total number of HIV-infected people in Thailand was fourteen times smaller than it would have been without the behavioral changes. As a result, the cost to treat all of Thailand's AIDS patients in the subsequent decade would be $18.6 billion less than without the behavioral changes. By spending $434 million to save $18.6 billion, Thailand achieved a benefit–cost ratio of forty-three to one, perhaps one of the highest computed for a government investment. In a world that has been spending $18 billion a year for AIDS treatment in low-income countries, donors would be irrational not to spend a few million to achieve measurable reductions in the rates of new HIV infections and thereby reduce the future need for treatment.

As figure 2-5 shows, by 2030, reducing incidence by 15 percent annually will save $2.6 billion in treatment costs a year, enough to finance treatment for at least 3 million additional AIDS patients. Reducing incidence by a much more dramatic 25 percent per year will save $3.8 billion by 2030, increasing to $8.5 billion a year by 2050. These two prevention

FIGURE 2-5.   Effect of Reductions in HIV Incidence on Costs and Deaths

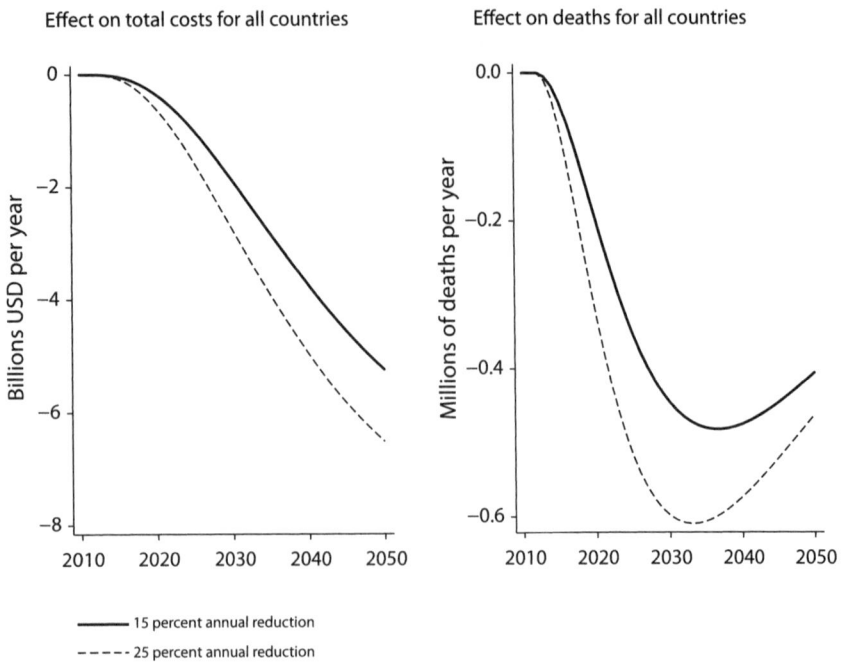

Source: Author's calculations.

scenarios also avert 600,000 and 800,000 deaths, respectively, with more averted from now to 2030 when the number of deaths would otherwise have crested, rather than later when people on treatment eventually succumb to the illness.

On a regional basis, table 2-3 shows that the benefits will be spread widely, with sub-Saharan Africa—the hardest-hit region—measuring the biggest gains if the rate of new cases is slowed from the current rate of decline of 5 percent per year to 15 percent or even 25 percent. Of the total cost saving of $2.6 billion from a 15 percent incidence rate, more than $1.9 billion would be saved in sub-Saharan Africa. Of the averted deaths, 427,000 out of 594,000 would be saved in sub-Saharan Africa.

These incidence reductions are easy to assume in a mathematical model but much harder to achieve in practice. However, the evidence of success with male circumcision and the success of well-established prevention techniques in the control groups of randomized controlled trials suggest that

TABLE 2-3. Better HIV Prevention: A Must for Sub-Saharan Africa

Region	Reduce incidence by 15 percent per year compared to 5 percent per year in baseline scenario		Reduce incidence by 25 percent per year compared to 5 percent per year in baseline scenario	
	Costs (thousands of US$)	Deaths	Costs (thousands of US$)	Deaths
East Asia and Pacific	−214,762	−51,128	−314,470	−65,994
Europe and Central Asia	−131,985	−35,340	−194,024	−45,592
Latin America and the Caribbean	−172,588	−23,270	−252,660	−29,936
Middle East and North Africa	−7,734	−3,987	−11,357	−5,158
South Asia	−146,831	−53,568	−215,891	−69,005
Sub-Saharan Africa	−1,963,796	−426,911	−2,879,985	−549,312
Total	−2,637,696	−594,204	−3,868,387	−764,997

Source: Author's calculations.

with sufficient effort and in the absence of political impediments, rates of incidence reduction of 15 percent or more are possible in Africa. Achieving incidence reductions of this magnitude can create fiscal space so that donors can contemplate expanding treatment access to a larger share of those in need.

CHAPTER 3

Sustaining and Leveraging
AIDS Treatment

The international donor community has succeeded in supporting a vast expansion of subsidized AIDS treatment, with service to a few thousand patients in 2003 growing to approximately 6 million in 2010. These patients are the beneficiaries of the first international entitlement program. Like its domestic counterparts, the AIDS treatment entitlement engenders dependency among its beneficiaries and restricts the flexibility of the donors and governments that assume its burden. This chapter presents original estimates of the magnitude of the future fiscal burden of AIDS treatment under alternative assumptions about treatment quality and expansion, then proposes policy options to harmonize the incentives among donors, recipient governments, and AIDS patients to sustain treatment quality while leveraging treatment demand for the prevention of future cases.

Donor-Supported AIDS Treatment: The First International Entitlement

At the 2005 summit meeting of the Group of Eight (G-8) in Gleneagles, Scotland, the assembled heads of state pledged "to develop and implement a package for HIV prevention, treatment and care, with the aim of as close as possible to universal access to treatment for all those who need it by 2010." They also promised, "We will work to meet the financing needs for HIV/AIDS."[1]

But when the International AIDS Society—a professional organization whose members include AIDS researchers and patients—convened in November 2009, it reflected on this commitment, stating, "Five years later, major donors and domestic governments appear to be *pulling back* on this commitment. While significant progress has been made toward expanding access to HIV prevention and treatment since 2005, the universal access goal is far from being met" (International AIDS Society 2009, 1, emphasis added).

The "significant progress" is the huge rise in the number of patients receiving subsidized AIDS treatment in low- and middle-income countries, mostly in sub-Saharan Africa. Of the 6 million patients receiving treatment by the end of 2010, about 3.2 million are supported by the U.S. President's Emergency Program for AIDS Relief (PEPFAR).[2] Thanks to this unprecedented international effort, the percentage of those needing and receiving treatment increased from less than 5 percent in 2003 to about 36 percent in 2009.

Unfortunately, although the term "universal access" has been defined in many ways—ranging from 100 percent to 80 percent coverage—all observers agree that 36 percent falls far short of that goal. Complicating matters, the World Health Organization (WHO) recently announced new guidelines that increased by 44 percent the number of people defined as "needing treatment," thus reducing the coverage rate from a hopeful 52 percent to a dismal 36 percent.[3] The attempt to provide treatment to all who need it looks more and more like the labor of Sisyphus, to whom the Greek gods set the task of pushing a boulder to the top of a hill, only to see it roll back to the bottom each time it got close.

But just when it seems that AIDS treatment requires even more funding if it is to reach all those in need, donors indeed are "pulling back" from their 2005 universal treatment commitment. Consider the case of PEPFAR. The bill to reauthorize the program passed Congress in 2008, before the end of President Bush's second term. That bill authorized $63 billion in new spending from 2009 through 2014, of which $39 billion is for HIV/AIDS treatment. Figure 3-1 shows the growth of PEPFAR funding for AIDS as enacted by Congress from 2004 through 2010 and as requested by the Obama administration for 2011. The uppermost line shows the total amount for bilateral AIDS support. The second line displays the minimum amount that Congress required PEPFAR to spend on AIDS treatment.[4] The rapid growth of U.S. funding for AIDS—at about 25 percent per year through 2008—has halted since that date, and the minimum amount mandated for treatment

FIGURE 3-1. U.S. Funding for AIDS: Universal Treatment Is Not on Track

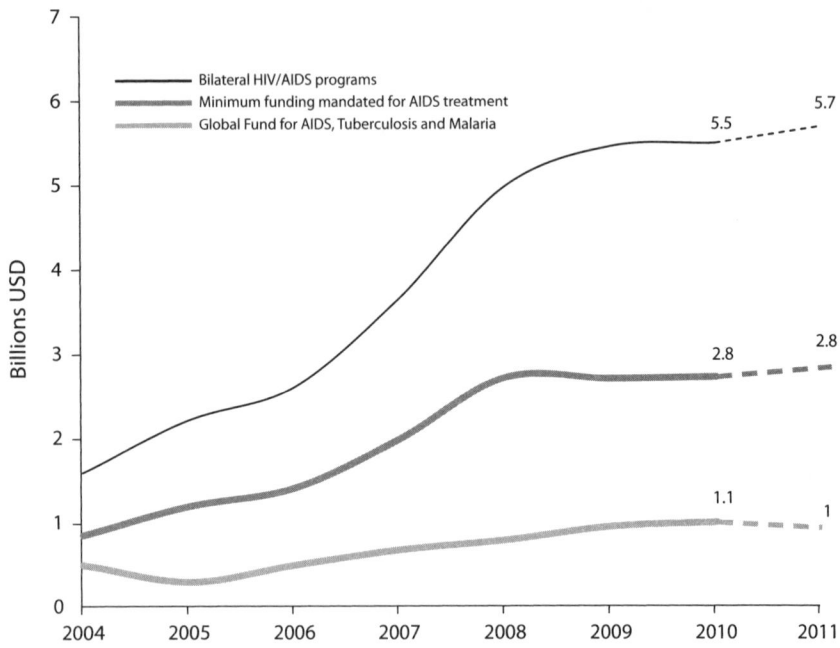

Source: U.S. President's Emergency Plan for AIDS Relief, "Making a difference: funding," fact sheet, October 2010, www. pepfar.gov/documents/organization/80161.pdf.

Note: Funding for 2004 through 2010 was enacted by Congress; funding for 2011 has been requested by the Obama administration.

has leveled. Other channels have not offset the plateau in United States bilateral funding for AIDS. The bottom line in figure 3-1 shows that U.S. funding for the Geneva-based, multilateral Global Fund for AIDS, Tuberculosis and Malaria, for example, also has flattened in recent years.

As a result of its scaled-back commitment, the United States draws a sharp distinction between patients whose antiretroviral therapy (ART) it is currently supporting and those with equal need who have not yet enrolled in treatment at a U.S.-supported site. Supporting the first group is an existing commitment. For patients not yet on treatment, the U.S. government will seek assurances that it alone will not bear all the future costs.

Illustrating this view, on April 11, 2010, Farah Stockman of the *Boston Globe* quoted a letter from the U.S. embassy in Kampala, Uganda, to PEPFAR-supported AIDS treatment facilities in that country as saying, "While the U.S. government is committed to continuing treatment for those individuals already enrolled ... funding for HIV programs is not expected to increase in the near future. As a result, PEPFAR Uganda cannot continue to support scale-up of antiretroviral treatment without a plan from the Government of Uganda on how these patients will be sustained." According to Ambassador Eric Goosby, the U.S. global AIDS coordinator and head of the PEPFAR program, the letter did not mean that U.S.-supported enrollment of new patients has stopped yet in Uganda. However, Stockman quotes him as saying, "People are struggling to find resources to honor the commitments we have made. . . . We're not at a cap point yet. If it gets worse, we'll have another discussion."[5]

To the extent that donors and their constituents agree that continued treatment of those already receiving it is sacrosanct, donor-financed support of AIDS treatment in low-income countries has created a new kind of international "entitlement." Although called an "emergency plan," the U.S. PEPFAR initiative has already endured longer than most emergency programs, and unless the United States either abandons or hands over its patients to other funders, PEPFAR is likely to persist longer than most foreign assistance projects. As *The Economist* notes,

> The problem with AIDS is that the more successful you are at treating it, the more you end up paying. That is because, unlike malaria and tuberculosis, it is incurable. Once someone is infected with HIV, the virus that causes it, they will end up requiring treatment for life. Good news for drugmakers, but bad news for both the poor who make up the overwhelming majority of the [33 million] people infected and for the taxpayers of the rich world who will be expected to find much of the money.[6]

Although the donors are not required by law to continue AIDS treatment, as would be true for domestic entitlements like the U.S. Social Security program, I believe that the international community and the voting public in democratic countries will constrain donors from dropping patients from treatment rolls. As the largest national donor, the United States will be seen as particularly accountable for sustaining this life-giving therapy, especially in the fifteen original PEPFAR focus countries.[7] Thus, AIDS treatment can be considered an entitlement, and all other types of international assistance financing, including for HIV prevention, become discretionary spending—that is, the money leftover in a budget after entitlements are funded (Over 2009b; Lyman and Wittels 2010).

From the donors' perspective, the downside of growing entitlements—in the absence of a very large increase in the total aid budget—is that the proportion of discretionary spending in donors' AIDS budgets will decline as donors place more patients on treatment. From the recipients' side, the downside of entitlements is dependency. Those who receive entitlements typically become dependent on them, and never more starkly than in the case of expensive life-giving drugs. The extreme form of aid dependency that AIDS treatment represents may have medium- and long-term negative repercussions.[8]

Because support for AIDS treatment converts foreign assistance from discretionary to entitlement spending, past treatment expenditure has already locked the United States and the other donor countries into a new aid paradigm. Advocates point to the unmet need for care and call for ever-increasing funding levels.[9] To the extent that the international community heeds the advocates' call for more resources, entitlement spending will greatly increase in the next few years. The increase will be absolute and, unless total assistance expands at the same phenomenal rate, as a share of total assistance.

Are voting taxpayers of the United States and other industrial countries ready for this new entitlement paradigm? Growing funding for AIDS treatment suggests this possibility. But there is reason for concern. Historically, when budgets expand less quickly than planned, growing entitlements often squeeze out discretionary programs. In the case of AIDS funding, the $50 billion a year requested by UNAIDS (The Joint United Nations Program on HIV/AIDS) from all donors to meet universal access to treatment and prevention could squeeze out spending on all eight of the United Nations Millennium Development Goals, which are aimed at boosting living standards worldwide.[10]

In the first chapter in this book, I propose a new framework for addressing the AIDS epidemic, which I call the AIDS transition. I define the AIDS transition as a dynamic process that preserves recently achieved mortality reductions while lowering the number of new infections even further so that the total number of people living with HIV/AIDS diminishes.

In this chapter, I discuss policy options for AIDS treatment that can sustain current patients on treatment while at the same time hastening the AIDS transition. In conformity with the view that current patients are entitled to continued treatment, none of the scenarios considers the possibility of reducing support for them. However, many other options are on the table. I project the cost of a range of new patient recruitment options, from enrolling no new patients to recruiting 80 percent of those in need according to the new WHO guidelines. I also contrast the cost of a policy that offers only the less expensive first-line therapy to the cost of a policy that puts patients on second-line therapy when first-line fails. And I show how a general move to initiate each patient's treatment earlier in the course of the illness has benefits but also significant costs. In a world of scarce financial resources, all these options involve trade-offs between cost savings and years of healthy life for the patients. While the calculations presented cannot determine how to choose among the alternative policies, they can elucidate the foregone opportunities implied by any choice and thus help policymakers and their constituencies choose wisely.

AIDS Treatment Successes and Failures

Several influential players have contributed to increase the number of people in low- and middle-income countries receiving ART from less than 100,000 in 2003 to approximately 6 million in 2010. Among those most responsible for this dramatic change are President Jacques Chirac of France and President George W. Bush of the United States.

From 1981, when the human immunodeficiency virus was discovered and identified as the cause of AIDS, until 1997, AIDS treatment was considered far too ineffective, complicated, and costly for governments or donors to fund in low- or even in middle-income countries. For example, in 1988, one year after the first antiretroviral drug, AZT, had been patented and before it was widely available, a global review of the cost of AIDS treatment found that a single patient-year of treatment cost $15,800 in Australia, $21,000 in France, $40,200 in Germany, $13,400–$46,000 in the United Kingdom, and $19,000–$147,000 in the United States—and rarely gave the patient more than a few months of healthy life (Scitovsky and Over 1988). In subsequent years, as medical research introduced new classes of drugs to directly attack the HIV retrovirus and the medical community accepted "triple-drug therapy," the effectiveness of treatment dramatically improved, while its potential cost rose. In the mid-1990s, the government of Thailand evaluated the cost-effectiveness of the new therapeutic combinations and concluded that "providing free antiretroviral therapy for symptomatic HIV infection, even with cost sharing, was unaffordable for both the public sector and the majority of patients" (van Praag and Perriens 1996, 440; see also Prescott 1997).

Writing in 1996 and 1997 on the priorities for government and donor intervention in the AIDS epidemic, World Bank economist Martha Ainsworth and I recognized the human tragedy unfolding as AIDS deaths climbed in AIDS-affected countries. But we were persuaded that given the high costs and still-limited effectiveness of ART, spending $10,000–$20,000 per patient-year on treatment would alleviate much less of that tragedy than would the same resources spent on prevention (Ainsworth and Over 1997). We hoped that donors and governments would use our book's argument for a dramatic increase in the most cost-effective types of HIV prevention to invigorate prevention efforts, especially in Africa. To that end, we launched our book during the opening session at the 1997 African AIDS conference, which was held that November in Abidjan, Côte d'Ivoire.

We received a bracing lesson there on the politics of AIDS treatment. President Chirac made a surprise appearance to give the keynote address, which immediately preceded our session. The contrast between his message and ours could not have been starker. While making only passing reference to the need for HIV prevention, President Chirac used his talk to issue a clarion call for donor funding of AIDS treatment and proposed the first global AIDS treatment initiative.[11]

Neither donors nor governments immediately responded to Chirac's proposal. Indeed, the European Commission, the World Bank, and the U.S. Agency for International Development all continued to emphasize prevention, though without scaling up to full coverage of high-risk populations as Ainsworth and I had recommended. However, in retrospect, Chirac's proposal is the historical precursor of subsequent much more successful efforts to expand AIDS treatment.

With President Bush's 2003 State of the Union address, the United States began a process that led to the creation of PEPFAR. While PEPFAR's objectives included treatment, prevention, and care, the political emphasis and the difficulties of measuring the achievement of these last two led to a focus on expanding AIDS treatment. By the end of Bush's presidency in December 2008, PEPFAR was reporting that it directly or indirectly supported approximately 3 million people on ART, and during 2008, another 1 million were added. As figure 3-2 shows, most of the 3.2 million people whose treatment PEPFAR directly supports reside in sub-Saharan Africa. Although the percentages of people infected are much smaller in Asia than in many African countries, the populations of China and India are so large that initial expansion of treatment there also contributes many people to the worldwide total.

While these achievements have been prodigious, few countries are managing to absorb a large percentage of all who need treatment into their treatment programs. In fact, as figure 3-3 shows, fewer than twenty of the world's low- and middle-income countries have achieved access—defined as the ratio of those on treatment to those needing treatment—of 80 percent or above. All the rest are reaching a minority of patients that need treatment. On a regional basis, countries with at least 80 percent access include two in East Asia and the Pacific, eight in Europe and Central Asia, three in Latin America and the Caribbean, five in the Middle East and North Africa, two in South Asia, and two in sub-Saharan Africa. However, most of these are small countries. Of the countries with more than 1,500 people needing treatment, only Chile, Costa Rica, and Namibia have managed to treat more than 80 percent of those in need. In all six regions, the majority of countries fall well behind these top performers.

What is each country's rate of treatment uptake—that is, the ratio of the number who are newly recruited during a year divided by the gap between those currently under treatment and the total needing it that year? This measure, which is a more dynamic way of viewing treatment success, captures the ability of a country program to absorb new patients as fast as people are developing the need for treatment.[12] As figure 3-4 shows, here, too, developing countries are split into two groups, with most at the low end. In sub-Saharan Africa in 2009, three-quarters of the countries were unable to extend treatment to half those in need according to UNAIDS' more conservative 2006 guidelines. And most of the good performers again are countries with small AIDS burdens (with the same few exceptions of Chile, Costa Rica, and Namibia).

Thus the complement to the optimistic story of increasing numbers of people on treatment is the increasing amount of unmet need—essentially a death sentence for those left untreated. People with AIDS usually start showing symptoms nine to eleven years from HIV infection (eART-linc 2008). But once symptoms appear, half of those who go untreated will die within a year, and almost all will die within three years. PEPFAR and its partners succeeded in slowing the growth of unmet need but not yet in reducing it in the world at large. This current and projected future persistence of unmet need despite the enormous effort and resources spent on treatment is one sign that donors and governments need to shift the policy objective from treatment access to the achievement of an AIDS transition.

Indicators of the Quality of Treatment

The expansion of the numbers on treatment is one measure of treatment success; the survival of people on treatment is another. How well have treatment programs been able to prolong the lives of those who begin treatment?

Although the ART drugs currently used by poor patients in low-income countries are far superior to those available a few years ago, achieving sustained health benefits from ART remains a substantial challenge to the health care provider and the patient. ART drugs must be taken for the

FIGURE 3-2. Cumulative Number of People Receiving Antiretroviral Therapy from Programs Supported by the U.S. President's Emergency Plan for AIDS Relief as of September 20, 2009

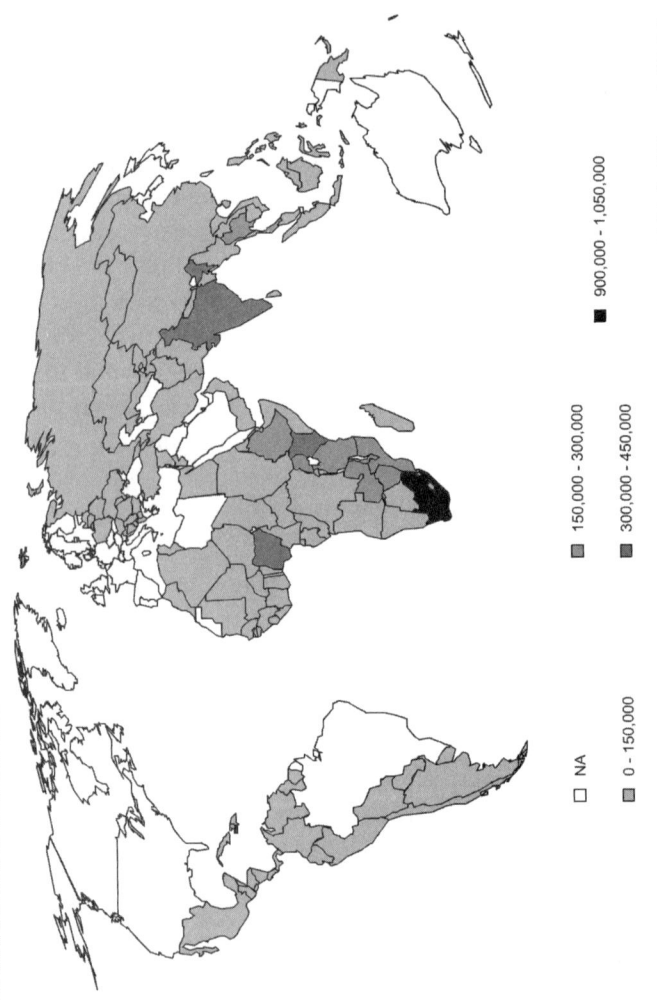

☐ NA

☐ 0 - 150,000

☐ 150,000 - 300,000

☐ 300,000 - 450,000

■ 900,000 - 1,050,000

Source: Henry J. Kaiser Family Foundation, "Reported number of people receiving antiretroviral therapy 2009" (globalhealthfacts.org). This information was reprinted with permission from the Henry J. Kaiser Family Foundation, a nonprofit private operating foundation, based in Menlo Park, California, dedicated to producing and communicating the best possible analysis and information on health issues.

FIGURE 3-3. Distribution of Low- and Middle-Income Countries by the Ratio of Those on Treatment to Those Needing Treatment

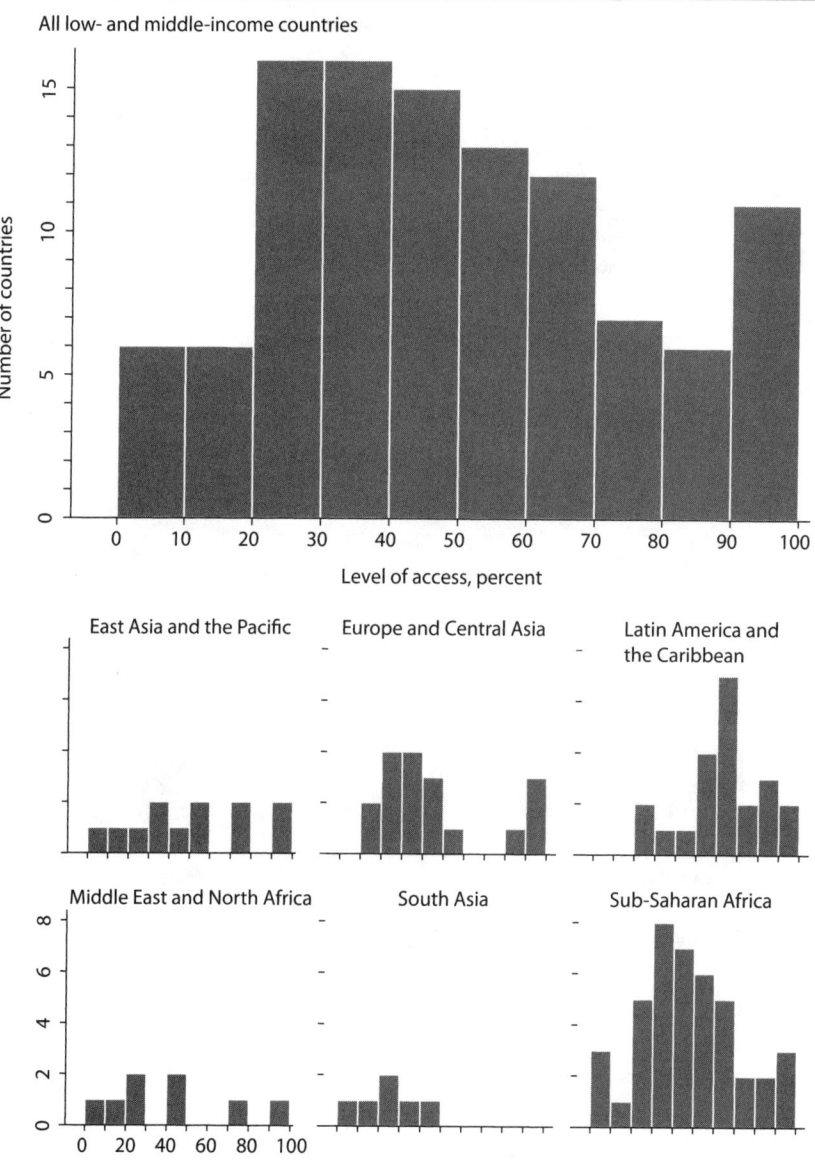

Note: Level of access is defined as the percentage of those needing treatment who receive treatment.

Source: Author's construction based on data from WHO, UNAIDS, and UNICEF 2009.

FIGURE 3-4. Distribution of Low- and Middle-Income Countries by Annual Uptake Rates for AIDS Treatment

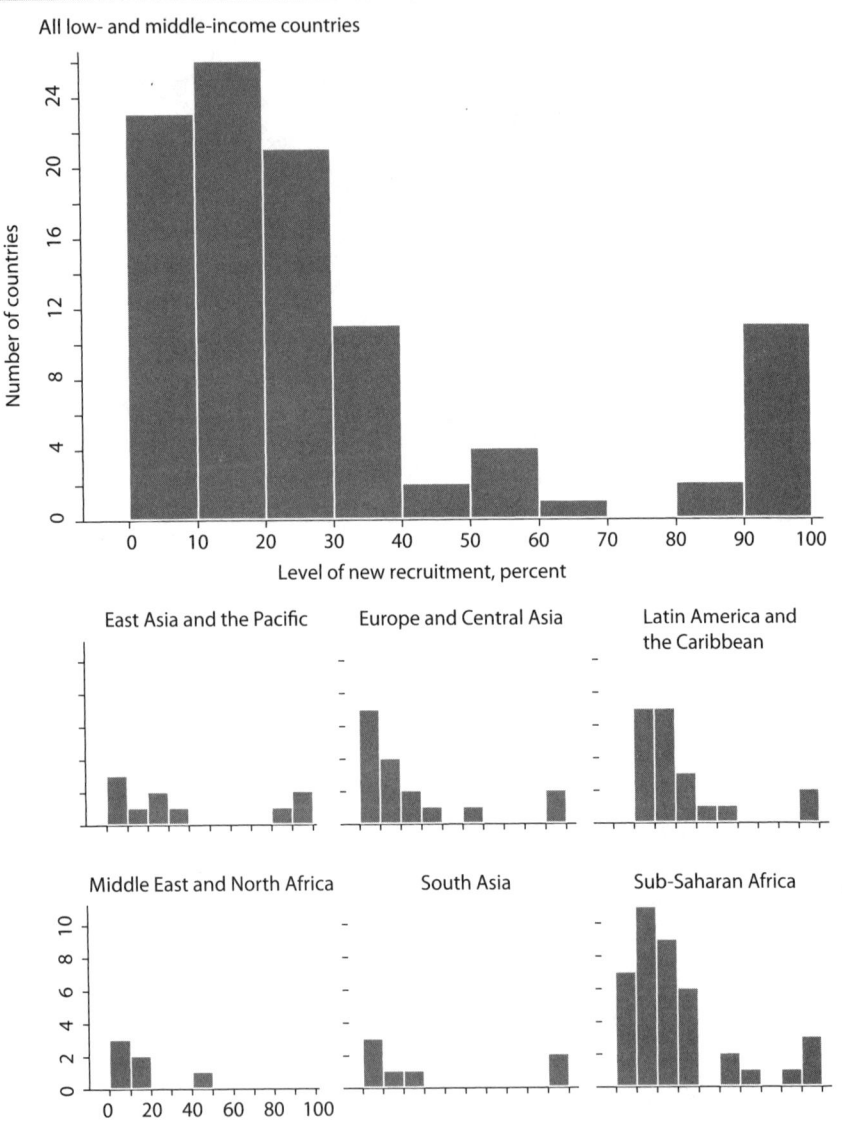

Note: Level of new recruitment is defined as the number of people who begin treatment in a year expressed as a percentage of those who need treatment but had not yet received it.

Source: Author's construction based on data from WHO, UNAIDS, and UNICEF 2009.

duration of the patient's life, once, twice, or more frequently each day, at specific times in relation to the consumption of food or liquids. Failure to adhere closely to the prescribed timing and dosages leads to the patient's development of a drug-resistant strain of HIV. Within months, the treatment will fail and the patient either will die or shift to a new and typically much more expensive drug combination. ART drugs have noxious side effects, such as diarrhea, indigestion, or worse for varying proportions of patients. These sometimes recede after a few months of treatment but can then reappear and prevent patients' necessary adherence to the treatment.[13] Socioeconomic obstacles to patient adherence include cultural and employer acceptance of AIDS, distance between the patient's home and the treatment facility, cost and availability of transportation, user fees at the health facility, and compensation for "treatment buddies" or other support personnel.

In view of the challenge that ART adherence represents, how well have ART programs done? This question is harder to answer than it might seem, for two reasons. First, in the early years of implementation, treatment programs have focused more on expanding access than on patient retention. Thus, they have neither reported nor always kept track of the information required to measure ART patient retention. This failure is perhaps understandable during the early years of such a novel and difficult initiative.

Second, even with good record keeping, clinics have difficulty knowing whether a patient who stops coming has failed treatment or simply changed treatment providers. Prior to the push to expand ART, few providers in these countries had either the training or the resources to systematically track patients suffering from other chronic illnesses, like diabetes or high blood pressure. So the need to track ART patients required providers to develop follow-up and outreach systems from scratch for this class of illnesses.

Given these difficulties, a conservative approach is to focus on patient retention as a measure of the quality of treatment programs. In response to a survey distributed by UNAIDS, sixty-one countries reported the number of patients remaining in treatment at twelve, twenty-four, thirty-six, and forty-eight months after treatment initiation. Figure 3-5 shows that only countries in the Middle East and North African region, where there are very few patients, reported more than 80 percent retention after twenty-four months. For sub-Saharan African countries—along with East, South, and Southeast Asian countries—retention at twenty-four months was less than 70 percent. Reviews of the literature on retention often point to the first six to twelve months as the critical period in a patient's treatment, during which ART treatment programs lose somewhere between 10 and 30 percent of patients (Rosen, Fox, and Gill 2007; Fox and Rosen 2010;

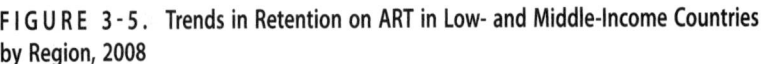

FIGURE 3-5. Trends in Retention on ART in Low- and Middle-Income Countries by Region, 2008

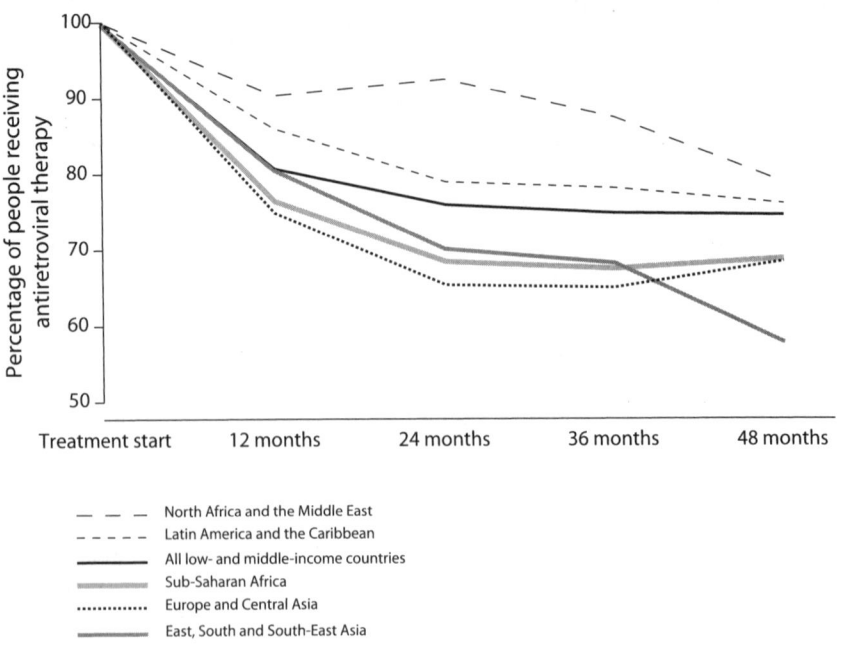

Source: WHO, UNAIDS, and UNICEF 2009, Figure 4.5.

and Wester and others 2009). But figure 3-5 leads to a more pessimistic assessment, suggesting that retention typically continues to drop for two full years before leveling off to a more moderate rate.

Treatment programs will be under constant pressure to spread resources more thinly so as to enroll a larger number of patients while accepting lower patient-retention rates. I argue that low-income countries with multiple health threats cannot afford to spend scarce public health system resources on ART programs with low patient-retention rates. Thus, an urgent question of operations research is how any given treatment budget can be allocated to maximize patient retention in AIDS treatment programs.

Foreign Assistance for AIDS Treatment

Given the huge resources raised for HIV/AIDS in recent years, am I unduly pessimistic to even worry about future funding? A look at the historical trend of health aid in general, and AIDS in particular, suggests the answer is no.

Since 1990 official development assistance for health-related objectives has grown rapidly, at a compound rate of 8 percent a year (Ravishankar and others 2009). The portion of total health assistance allocated to HIV/AIDS has grown even faster, at an average rate of about 20 percent a year. This extremely rapid rise in HIV/AIDS funding has fueled the growth in the numbers of people receiving ART and greatly expanded the scope of other HIV/AIDS interventions, including HIV prevention and support for orphans and vulnerable children. But can it, or even should it, continue at such a high growth rate in the coming years?

An examination of the growth trend of total funding for HIV/AIDS reveals a surprising discontinuity in its rate of increase. The data suggest that before 1999 the growth of HIV/AIDS spending in constant 2007 dollars was steady at about 13 percent per year. This growth rate was about twice as fast as the 5.8 percent growth of non-HIV/AIDS health assistance during that period and, if continued, would have increased steadily the share of HIV/AIDS in total health official development assistance. But then in 1999, the rate of growth of HIV/AIDS funding more than doubled, from 13 to 28 percent per year, an accelerated rate that continued until the deceleration of PEPFAR funding that began after 2008.[14] At the same time, the rate of growth of non-health assistance remained unchanged.[15]

What could account for the dramatic acceleration in donor assistance for HIV/AIDS in comparison to all other health problems? The disaggregation of HIV/AIDS assistance by donor makes clear that the increased growth in 2000 owed to increased contributions from several larger donors but not from the United States (Ravishankar and others 2009, figure 29). The World Bank increased its allocation to HIV/AIDS in 1999 and then followed by launching its Multi-Country AIDS Program in September 2000. The Bill and Melinda Gates Foundation started spending on HIV/AIDS in 2000. UNAIDS funding also jumped upward in that year. U.S. spending did not increase substantially until 2002 and then accelerated in 2004, when the U.S. PEPFAR program kicked in. U.K. spending took its first large jump in HIV/AIDS assistance in 2004. And the Global Fund for AIDS, Tuberculosis and Malaria began disbursing funds in 2003, greatly increasing its disbursements in 2004.

Looked at in aggregate, the trend since 1999 in HIV/AIDS assistance is remarkably smooth. All the major donors have played their roles, some increasing their funding one year and others another year, so that on average across all donors and recipients, the trend has been one of constant growth at 28 percent a year. Over this period, the U.S. government's contribution has grown but no more rapidly than that of other donors. The

FIGURE 3-6. Domestic and Foreign Sources of AIDS Funding in Low- and Middle-Income Countries, 2005–08

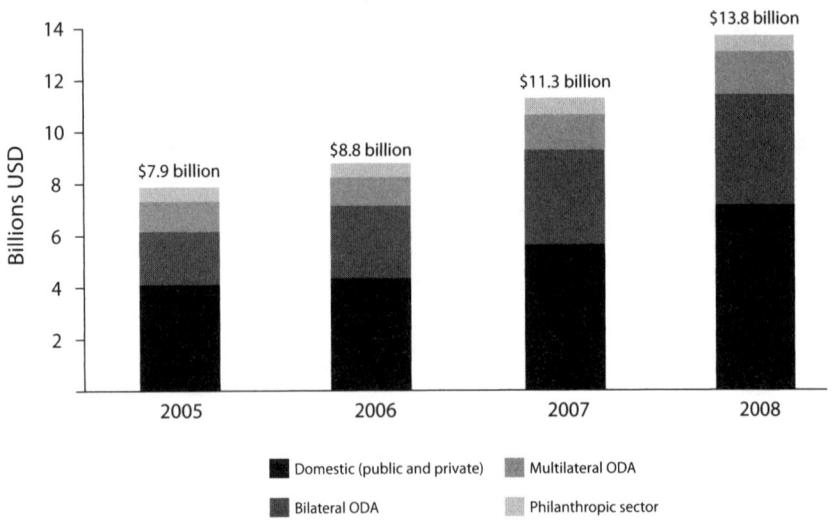

Source: WHO, UNAIDS, and UNICEF 2009.
Note: ODA = official development assistance.

result has been that the United States has maintained its share of total HIV/AIDS funding at slightly less than 50 percent throughout this historical period.

Furthermore, as figure 3-6 shows, in recent years domestic spending has kept pace with donor spending, which accounts for about half of total AIDS expenditures. Although a breakdown of domestic funding between AIDS treatment and HIV prevention is not available, it seems likely that middle-income countries financed more than half of AIDS treatment through relatively developed health insurance and financing systems, while poorer countries probably depended more on donors.

This high level of AIDS assistance is unlikely to continue, as the stage seems set for a slowdown in the growth of AIDS assistance. The World Bank has discontinued its special funding for AIDS. The Global Fund for AIDS, Tuberculosis and Malaria is complaining of funding shortfalls. And the United States first moved to slow the growth of AIDS funding with the 2008 PEPFAR reauthorization bill and then folded AIDS into its new Global Health Initiative in 2009–2010. In her first major policy speech on foreign assistance in January 2010, Secretary of State Hillary Clinton said,

One of our country's most notable successes in development is PEP-FAR, which has helped more than 2.4 million people with HIV receive life-saving antiretroviral medications. Now PEPFAR will be the cornerstone of our new Global Health Initiative. We will invest $63 billion over the next six years to help our partners improve their health systems and provide the care their people need, *rather than* rely on donors to keep a fraction of their population healthy while the rest go with hardly any care (emphasis added).[16]

Her speech suggests that U.S. health assistance should avoid focusing too narrowly on increasing the numbers of AIDS patients who benefit from ART support, instead strengthening recipient countries' ability to serve a broader range of patients. Her words imply that PEPFAR's role in the entire U.S. health assistance edifice should and will diminish over time as health-sector aid is rebalanced.

Secretary Clinton's speech unfortunately also suggests that the United States is considering reneging on the implicit lifetime entitlement it had already granted to the 2.4 million people in 24 low- and middle-income countries now on U.S.-funded AIDS treatment. I doubt that Secretary Clinton meant to wave that red flag, given that such a decision would contradict the objectives announced by PEPFAR on December 1, 2009, to respect the entitlement and add at least another 1.6 million people to the U.S.-supported treatment rolls by the year 2014. By September 2010 PEPFAR had added another 800,000 to its treatment rolls for a total of 3.2 million supported patients, but this rate of increase is 20 percent less than it had been in the previous year. While PEPFAR now seems likely to surpass its target of 4 million patients supported by the year 2014, the accumulating burden of patients already on treatment combined with the apparent diminished enthusiasm of the newly elected Congress to support entitlements at home or abroad suggests that fewer patients will be added to treatment rolls in future years.

The Reduction in the Cost of Treating One AIDS Patient

A more clear-cut success in the treatment of HIV/AIDS is its decreasing cost per person. Effective AIDS treatment began in 1993 with the introduction of AZT, the first drug that could slow HIV reproduction. But as discussed, treatment with an antiviral drug and drugs for the attendant opportunistic illnesses cost as much as $100,000 per year and was only available in high-income countries (Scitovsky and Over 1988). Furthermore, it soon became apparent that treatment with the single antiviral would help a patient for only a limited number of years before the virus developed resistance to that drug and would again spread within the body with fatal results.[17] In response medical researchers developed the concept of combination therapy or triple-drug therapy, which greatly slowed the development of drug resistance in the individual patient. However, as discussed, these more effective combination therapy regimes also are more complex for the doctors and patients—and more expensive as well. By 1997 the cost of triple-drug ART averaged $20,000 per patient-year, with only occasional lower-price deals available for a few middle-income countries, such as Thailand and Brazil, that bargained sufficiently forcefully with the drug firms (Ainsworth and Over 1997). That was the year when President Chirac proposed extending ART to all, an objective that seemed quixotic because of the cost per patient and the numbers in need.

Since that time, AIDS treatment has improved remarkably in quality while the cost per patient-year has continued to fall. In the late 1990s and the early 2000s, quality improvements stemmed from scientific breakthroughs in understanding the biology of the virus and better health service delivery systems for ART.

Increasing the availability of the drugs, Indian pharmaceutical firms entered into the production and distribution of generic versions of branded ART drugs—a trend that the multinational firms holding the patents for those drugs and the U.S. government at first vigorously opposed. Pressure by AIDS advocates and a coalition of nongovernmental organizations led by the Clinton Foundation helped the WHO promote the use of these generic drugs, and in 2006, PEPFAR switched to the generics (Holmes and others 2010).

The result of these various pressures on drug prices has been dramatic reductions over the last ten years of as much as 90 percent in the annual cost in the poorest countries of drugs required for ART. Figure 3-7 shows that drug prices continued to fall between 2006 and 2009 but at a decreasing rate. The two panels of figure 3-7 show the trends over time in the annual cost for the most widely used combinations of first-line (panel a) and second-line (panel b) treatments within low-income countries. In panel a, the annual cost of the most-used combination on the left declined by almost 50 percent.[18] The second and third combinations in panel a were used by 22 and 19 percent patients, respectively, and their annual costs declined by even more than 50 percent. Similar patterns of decline are apparent in panel b describing annual drug costs on second-line treatment in the same countries.[19]

However, after years of decline, drug prices now seem to be stabilizing. According to the WHO, UNAIDS, and UNICEF (2010, 70–72), between 2008 and 2009, the weighted median price of the six most widely used first-line regimens declined only 3 percent in low-income countries and 13 percent in the lower-middle-income countries, and it actually increased by 21 percent in the upper-middle-income countries. The organizations attribute the increase in the higher-income countries to their adoption of the newer, less toxic drug tenofovir disoproxil fumarate in first-line regimes (WHO, UNAIDS, and UNICEF 2010, 72). When poorer countries begin to make the same substitution, their annual costs also will rise unless offset by further price reductions.

What will be the average cost of a patient-year of treatment in the years ahead? The statistical analysis of the variation of total AIDS expenditures across countries and over the three years reveals that the average cost of a patient-year of treatment increases with the country's level of income but declines with the total number of enrolled patients. Average costs also declined between 2005 and 2006 but not between 2006 and 2007. Appendix A explains how one can use this aggregate relationship to estimate the average cost of first-line AIDS treatment for future years, assuming that the affected countries grow at rates predicted by the World Bank and allowing average cost to decline with any projected increase in the number of ART patients. The average total cost of first-line treatment for a country with 25,000 first-line patients is presented in row h of table 3-1. It varies from $296 per patient-year for a country with an income of $460 per capita to $1,690 for a country with an income of $5,430 per capita.

To project the impact of a gradual shift toward second-line treatment, I extract the first-line drug costs from the estimated total cost and replace them with projected second-line drug costs. To be sure this procedure is internally consistent, I first decompose average total cost into two components, the average variable cost and the average fixed cost. I estimate the average variable cost from the bottom up, by adding an estimated annual cost of first-line drugs (which varies with the country's income) to estimated in-patient and out-patient costs per patient-year, arriving at the figures in row e of table 3-1. I subtract average variable cost from average total cost, arriving at an estimate of average fixed cost, which is in row h of table 3-1. This calculation suggests that fixed costs are a large percentage of total costs, ranging from 43 percent for a low-income country to 80 percent for an upper-middle-income country.

Then I proceed to construct second-line costs. I assume that the fixed cost and the non-drug elements of the variable cost remain the same as for

FIGURE 3-7. The Median Annual Price of Antiretroviral Treatments in Low-Income Countries, 2006–09

Panel A. First-line treatments

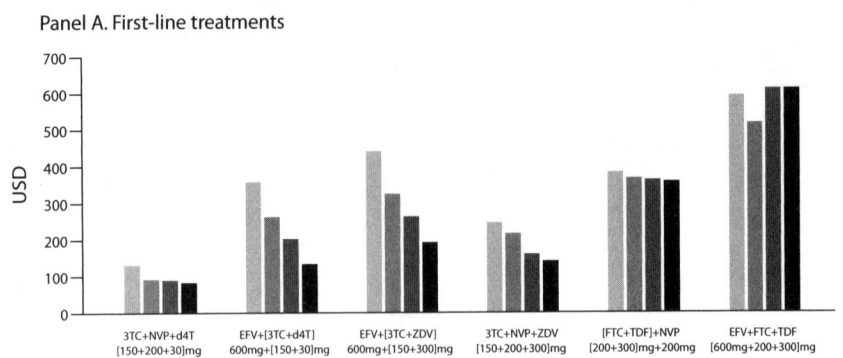

Panel B. Second-line treatments

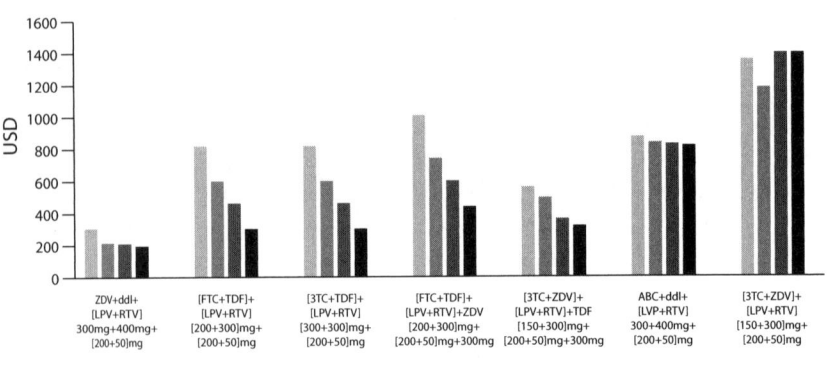

■ 2006 ■ 2007 ■ 2008 ■ 2009

Source: Adapted from WHO, UNAIDS, and UNICEF 2010, figures 4-10 and 4-12.
Note: ZDV = Zidovudine; ddI = didanosine; LPV=lopinavir + ritonavir; RTV=ritonavir; mg = milligrams; FTC = emtricitabine; TDF = tenofovir disoproxil/fumarate; 3TC = lamivudine; ABC = abacavir.

first-line therapy. By adding rows b, c, and d of table 3-1, I compute the average variable cost for second-line therapy, presented in row f of the table. Average total cost of second-line therapy is then just the sum of rows f and g. Presented in row i of table 3-1, the average total cost of second-line therapy varies from $1,151 per patient year in the low-income country to $3,645 per patient year in the upper-middle-income country.

So what is the bottom line? Overall the effects of economic growth and treatment scale-up are likely to balance out so that average costs for AIDS treatment will be relatively stable going forward. I now use these projec-

TABLE 3-1. Average Annual Cost per Enrolled Patient and Cost Components of AIDS Treatment for Countries Enrolling 25,000 Patients at Three Different Income Levels, 2007

Annual cost components	Low-income country ($460 per capita)	Lower-middle-income country ($2,000 per capita)	Upper-middle-income country ($5,430 per capita)
a. First-line drugs	$148	$209	$234
b. Second-line drugs	$1,003	$1,629	$2,189
c. Inpatient days (1.56)	$16.30	$39.36	$71.77
d. Outpatient visits (9.5)	$4.96	$13.79	$27.61
e. Average variable cost: first-line therapy (rows a + c + d)	$169	$262	$333
f. Average variable cost: second-line therapy (rows b + c + d)	$1,024	$1,682	$2,288
g. Average fixed cost (assuming 25,000 patients)	$127	$573	$1,357
h. Average total cost (first-line therapy) (rows e + g)	$296	$835	$1,690
i. Average total cost (second-line therapy) (rows f + g)	$1,151	$2,255	$3,645

Sources: Costs of first- and second-line drugs are interpolated to the specified income level from WHO, UNAIDS, and UNICEF 2009. Average number of inpatient and outpatient days per AIDS patient per year (1.56 and 9.5 in rows c and d) are from personal communication with John Stover of the Futures Institute, March 2010. Average total cost of first-line therapy (row h) is estimated by the author from data on total expenditure on ART, total patients on ART, and gross national income per person. See Appendix A for details.

tions of average fixed costs to show how countries' AIDS policy choices affect the future fiscal burden that they and their donors will shoulder.

The Future Fiscal Burden of Treatment

Only a few years ago, the WHO championed the idea that the world should strive to provide universal access to AIDS treatment for all who need it, and it still references this goal in the title of recent reports on AIDS (WHO, UNAIDS, and UNICEF 2007, 2009, 2010).[20] What would universal access cost and how plausible is it as an objective?

The Future Cost of AIDS Treatment

International donor subsidies to the cost of AIDS treatment in low-income countries are already large—in 2007, all donors together spent an estimated total of $5 billion on AIDS, of which about half was spent on treatment (Ravishankar and others 2009). This amount jumped to $7.7 billion in 2008 and then remained virtually constant at $7.6 billion for

FIGURE 3-8. Antiretroviral Therapy (ART): Number, Costs, and Entitlement with Universal Access, 2010–50

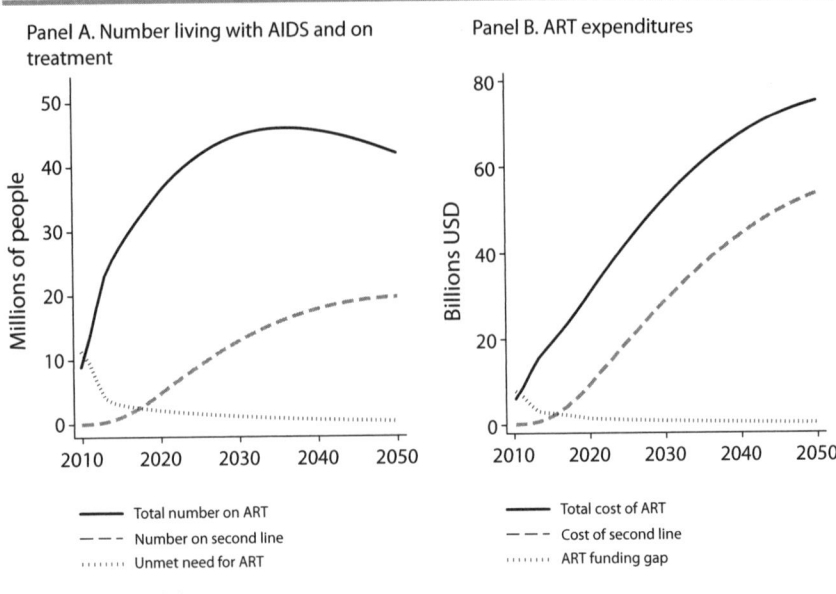

Panel A. Number living with AIDS and on treatment

Panel B. ART expenditures

Source: Author's calculations.

2009.[21] How much would it cost if the world opts for universal treatment—that is, if 80 percent of those in need receive treatment when they reach the WHO's new criterion for treatment of a CD4 count of 350 cells per milliliter? To calculate this figure, I project unit costs as described in table 3-1 and appendix A and assume that the number of new infections drops at 5 percent per year. As figure 3-8 shows, by the year 2030, the number of people on treatment will increase more than ten-fold to about 45 million, and the annual cost will rise by an even greater multiple to $50 billion (constant 2009 dollars).[22]

To gauge the magnitude of this sum, note first that it does not include any expenditure on other objectives of HIV/AIDS policy, such as HIV prevention and care for those orphaned or widowed by the disease. It is twice the total value of all U.S. foreign assistance in 2007, which was about $26 billion, including aid to Afghanistan, Egypt, and Israel (Radelet, Abarcar, and Schutte 2009). And it is almost half the total amount of foreign assistance by all donors in 2007, which was $103.5 billion.[23] Moreover, if total foreign assistance continues to grow at about 3 percent per year in real terms (which is optimistic given that this would be faster than the projected growth of the high-income countries' GDP) and only half the $50 billion must be funded by donors (as suggested by figure 3-6), reaching universal access under these assumptions would require that $25 billion of $180 billion in foreign assistance, or about one-seventh of the total, be spent on AIDS treatment.

Under these assumptions, the prodigious expenditure of about half a trillion dollars on AIDS treatment over the next twenty years would achieve the AIDS transition—because by the year 2032, the total number of new infections worldwide would fall from the current level of more than 2 million per year to about 715,000 per year, which would be slightly less than the number of deaths from AIDS that year. As a result, the number of people living with AIDS and the number on AIDS treatment would begin a slow decline but would remain above 40 million until the year 2050 and beyond (figure 3-8, panel a). Expenditures would continue to rise for another two decades, reaching $75 billion by the year 2050 (figure 3-8, panel b). In the absence of dramatic improvements in first-line therapy, by the year 2050 almost half of the patients will have failed this regimen and moved on to second-line drugs (figure 3-8, panel a)—or to even more expensive alternatives—consuming two-thirds of total treatment expenses (figure 3-8, panel b).

My goal is to present a vision of a faster AIDS transition, one that would sustain current AIDS entitlements and add to the treatment rolls while remaining affordable. To this end, suppose that HIV prevention becomes much more effective, so that the decline in new cases occurs at 15 percent per year instead of 5 percent per year. And suppose that the uptake percentage in each country will remain about the same as the uptake that has been achieved the last three years, with about 30 percent of those in need being added to treatment rolls each year—but in this case, the average CD4 count at ART initiation is 130 (consistent with recent experience).

Changing these assumptions decreases by two-thirds the number of people on treatment, which peaks in 2033 (figure 3-9, panel a). Although 30 percent of those needing treatment receive it each year, the total number on treatment eventually declines as the result of the natural life cycle of those on treatment, and the number of people living with HIV/AIDS declines steadily because of the declining incidence of new infections starting now. Total costs in 2030 are $21.4 billion instead of $50 billion, for a reduction of more than 50 percent (figure 3-9, panel b). Under this scenario, the number of new infections soon drops below the number of deaths.[24] The AIDS transition is within reach.

FIGURE 3-9. Antiretroviral Therapy (ART): Numbers, Costs, and Entitlement with 30 Percent Uptake, 2010–50

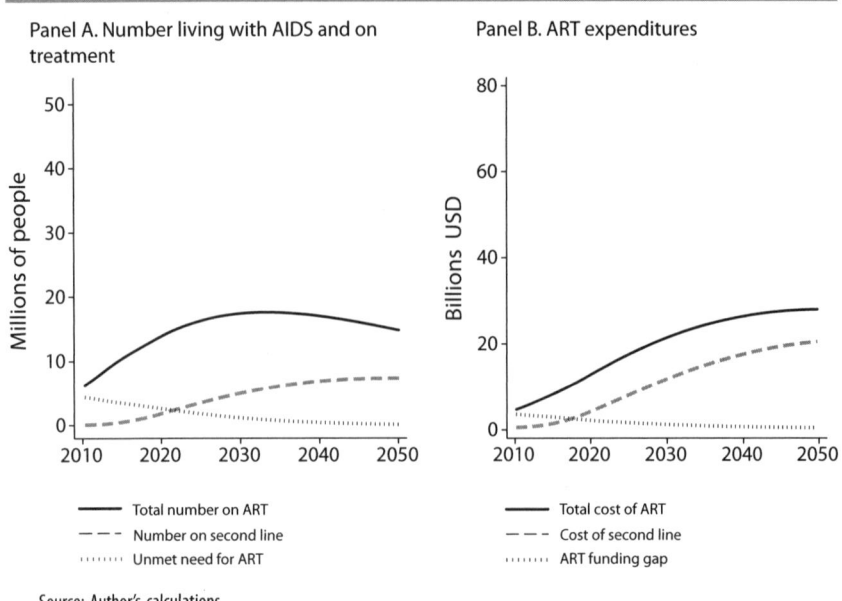

Source: Author's calculations.

Possible "Game-Changing" Shocks to Future Treatment Costs

The projection that the cost of offering universal access to AIDS treatment might hit $50 billion per year in 2030 and exceed $75 billion by 2050 is based on a large number of assumptions, about which reasonable people can disagree. Several are particularly crucial to the estimates of future costs. In this section, I discuss possible changes in government and donor policy that could alter those assumptions and thereby greatly increase or decrease future costs.

CHANGE IN RECRUITMENT THRESHOLD. On November 30, 2009, the WHO released revised guidelines recommending that patients begin treatment when their CD4 count reaches 350 rather than waiting until it drops to 200 (WHO 2009). But debate continues regarding whether low-income countries should adopt the new AIDS treatment guidelines or continue to prioritize recruitment at a CD4 count of 200. The existence of a health benefit is one side of the story, and a recent study provides convincing evidence that in resource-rich settings, beginning ART at 350 offers definite health advantages to the average person with HIV (When to Start Consortium and Sterne 2009). The other side of the story, however, is the cost of earlier treatment initiation, which increases because of the longer period of treatment. But how much costs will rise hinges on whether, and by how long, the patient's death is postponed. For policymakers, two key questions arise. How large will the cost increase be compared to the increased benefit? And when there are insufficient resources to cover the costs of all who need treatment at more advanced stages of the disease, how should policymakers weigh the use of resources for healthier people against the recruitment of a larger percentage of sicker people?

To better understand the trade-off involved in moving to an earlier CD4 count, consider the situation from the point of view of the PEPFAR program. On December 1, 2009, the White House announced a new five-year strategy for PEPFAR that aims to increase the number of patients PEPFAR directly supports on ART from the 2.4 million on treatment when the plan was announced to at least 4 million by 2014. PEPFAR managers can meet this goal in two ways that cost about the same: recruit earlier by starting HIV-infected people on treatment before they are very sick, as counseled by the new WHO guidelines, or expand access by directing the drugs to people who have been infected longer and are therefore sicker. The second choice seems the most humane and equitable: give drugs to the patients who need them most. However, because the prognosis of these patients is generally worse than that of people more recently infected, recruiting patients earlier in their illness actually averts more deaths.

Figure 3-10 helps visualize PEPFAR's dilemma by plotting various contours to show the trade-off between the annual rate of uptake of new patients (on the vertical axis) and the starting CD4 count at ART initiation (on the horizontal axis). The black curved line of figure 3-10 shows combinations of uptake rate and CD4 count at start of treatment that will achieve PEPFAR's goal of 4 million patients enrolled in 2014. The target number can be reached through late recruitment—for example, when the CD4 count is 100—provided the uptake rate is around 13 percent to replace the large number of patients who fail treatment. Alternatively the same number can be reached through early recruitment—for example, when the CD4 count is 350—with a lower uptake rate of 9 percent because the program would retain more patients until 2014. The gray curved line shows the combinations that will cost $11 billion in additional funding through 2014. The two sets of combinations are almost identical, reflecting the fact that all points on this frontier are produced with the same number of years of treatment.[25]

The diagonal lines in figure 3-10 show how expanding ART by either increasing annual uptake or recruiting earlier will reduce deaths. The lower

FIGURE 3-10. PEPFAR's Conundrum: Early Recruitment or Large Enrollment?

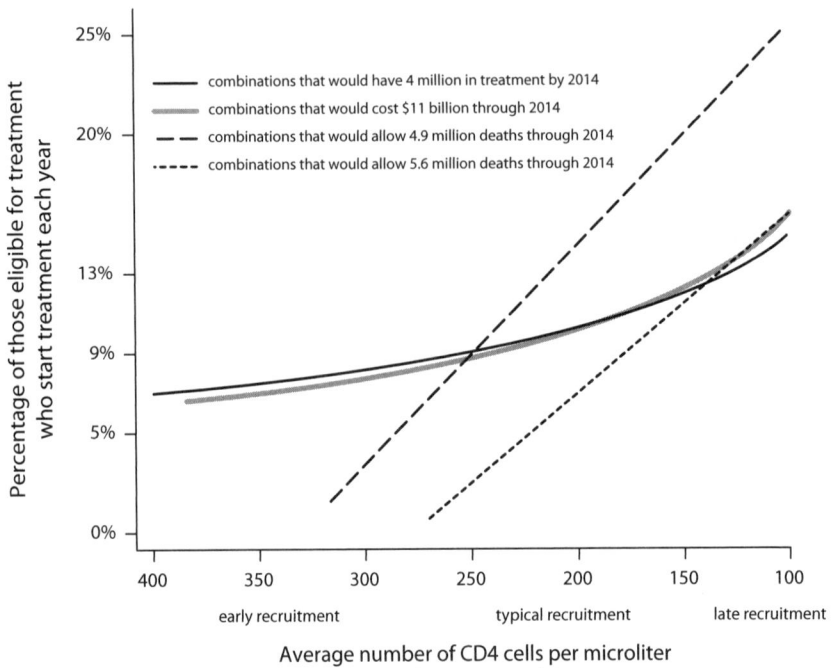

Source: Author's estimates as described in appendixes a and b.

of the two lines shows the combinations of uptake and recruitment threshold that will allow about 5.6 million AIDS deaths in these countries through 2014. The upper diagonal line shows the combinations that will allow about 4.9 million deaths. Thus a policy decision to move from any point on the lower line to any point on the upper line will postpone about 700,000 deaths.

Figure 3-10 allows comparison of the cost-effectiveness of the two alternative strategies: keeping the recruitment CD4 count at its current value of about 130 and raising it to 250.[26] Because the lines depicting equal number of deaths are steeper than the line depicting equal cost, moving from 130 to 250 costs no more but saves an additional 700,000 lives.

Thus, if the objective were to use the 4 million patient enrollment target and the associated budget to postpone as many deaths as possible beyond 2014, PEPFAR and its partners should favor a policy of lower access with early recruitment (a 9 percent uptake at a median CD4 count of 250) over higher access with continued late recruitment (a 13 percent uptake with median CD4 at initiation unchanged from 130). In terms of postponed deaths, early recruitment with lower uptake would be the more cost-effective policy.

However, this cost-effectiveness comparison is not sufficient to propose a blanket PEPFAR policy of preferring early recruitment to increased access. To begin with, in comparison to the ideal of universal access, even the less cost-effective annual uptake rate of 13 percent denies treatment each year to 87 percent of those who are eligible for it. While other sources of financing in these countries, including the Global Fund for AIDS, Tuberculosis and Malaria, national governments, domestic and international NGOs, and the patients themselves might together directly support another 1 or 2 million patients, perhaps increasing the uptake rate from 13 to 30 or even 40 percent, this would still leave many patients without care. Furthermore, the choice to allocate resources to earlier recruitment rather than increased access implies prioritizing relatively healthy HIV-positive patients for treatment over those with low CD4 counts who are in more desperate straits. These considerations are likely to convince many policymakers to prioritize access over early recruitment, regardless of the increased number of deaths.

These are tough choices with no easy answers. While PEPFAR may have a view about which point on the 4 million patient contour to aim for, I believe it would be unethical for any donor to impose the choice of any given point on this contour on other governments. The difficulty of this choice, and of other choices that involve trade-offs, underlines the importance of another theme of PEPFAR's new strategy—partnership in decision-making with the host country.

CHANGE IN THE COSTS OF DRUGS. As discussed above, in the past decade, substantial savings on drug costs have been achieved through increased competition from generic versions and bulk procurement agreements with the manufacturers of branded drugs. The Clinton Foundation has taken the lead in the negotiations that have achieved the price reductions of branded drugs. Given the foundation's role in achieving these historic price reductions, it is noteworthy that in a recent article proposing ways to bridge the resource gap in AIDS treatment, its chief executive officer points to pressures that might raise the cost per patient of first-line drugs. For example, a drug called stavudine, which costs $80 per patient-year, can be replaced with a drug with fewer side effects called tenofovir, which costs $200 per patient-year (Soni and Gupta 2009).

Furthermore, as Indian pharmaceutical firms are increasingly constrained by India's participation in the World Trade Organization's Trade-Related Aspects of Intellectual Property Rights (TRIPS) agreement to respect the patents of multinational pharmaceutical companies, they may compete less aggressively in the markets that supply low-income countries with these drugs. If this occurs, either the market share of less-expensive Indian generics might fall or their average prices might cease decreasing—or might even rise. Innovations in the design of drug-procurement mechanisms such as the WHO's recently developed Global Price Reporting Mechanism and the Department for International Development–funded Medicine Transparency Alliance may help reduce the prices of drugs in transactions between low-income countries and major donors. However, the opportunity for achieving dramatic additional price reductions on first-line drugs may be limited in the future

As for second-line drugs, UNAIDS recently reported that few patients in low- or middle-income countries currently are receiving this treatment with public resources. Data from the WHO's Global Price Reporting Mechanism show that the percentage of publicly funded patients in countries outside Latin America receiving second-line therapy has declined from 4 percent in 2006 to 2 percent in 2009. The decline in the proportion of patients on second-line treatment observed in the WHO's sample probably reflects the rapid increase in patients starting ART, almost all on first-line treatment. However, in the Americas, the WHO reports that the proportion receiving publicly funded second-line or so-called "salvage" therapy is about 16 percent, or about eight times as large as the proportion in the rest of the world (WHO, UNAIDS, and UNICEF 2010, 66). As treatment access expands, we can expect that patients will fail first-line treatment and need to move to second-line, placing additional pressure on AIDS treatment budgets (Soni and Gupta 2009).[27]

The bottom line is that while the cost per patient-year of second-line drugs may continue to fall in the future, as it has in the past few years, the pressures to slow or reverse reductions in first-line drug prices apply with equal force to second-line drugs. Thus, for future projections, I assume that first-line and second-line drug prices will remain constant.

INCREASED TASK-SHIFTING TO REDUCE CLINIC COSTS. Delegating routine AIDS treatment tasks that physicians previously performed to mid-level health care personnel can potentially improve efficiency and lower costs, without sacrificing quality. The United States has experimented with delegation in ambulatory medical care for decades, with a particular push immediately after the Vietnam War (Golladay and others 1976). But this strategy is limited when the mid-level personnel are insufficient in numbers or lack the training to take on ART tasks.

Some have attributed the lack of health care personnel in low-income countries to the exodus of skilled personnel in the search of higher incomes in richer countries, but others argue that an increase in the number of physicians from a given country who work abroad goes hand-in-hand with an increase in the number working at home. Take the case of Zambia, which has one of the worst AIDS epidemics in the world. The Zambian government has analyzed its health manpower shortage and concluded that to address its physician shortage at home, it must increase enrollment in its health-training institutions, which means increasing their capacity and attracting more students (Soni and Gupta 2009). As my colleague Michael Clemens (2007) has pointed out, a country is not likely to attract the most qualified students to its expanded health-training program if it attempts to limit mobility after graduation. By increasing its production of physicians and nurses and accepting that a proportion of them will emigrate, Zambia hopes to emulate other countries with strong health programs, such as South Africa, Mauritius, and Tunisia, which have many physicians abroad and at home.

Another constraint on task delegation is the scale of a medical practice. If the number of patients is small and each requires at least an occasional minute of the doctor's time, the most economical staff design is that of the solo practitioner. As the number of patients expands, opportunities emerge for health personnel to specialize and physicians to delegate an increasing share of their work. Indeed, specialization and delegation are two ways in which economies of scale can be realized.

RISING COSTS OF APPROACHING FULL COVERAGE. Discussions about scaling up AIDS treatment frequently assume that returns to scale will perpetually increase because unit costs of treatment will be ever lower. Recently, however, experts in the medical community have joined economists in warning that the advances in treatment so far obtained have been the low-hanging fruit; pursuing additional, more difficult advances could cause costs even to increase.

One reason that unit costs of treatment might rise dramatically would be the effort to extend treatment into smaller population centers. If important reductions in unit cost indeed are obtainable from increasing the number of patients served from a small to medium number, the converse would also be true: there will be diseconomies in building and operating the small-scale AIDS treatment centers that will be required to extend coverage outside the major urban centers of the developing world. The effort to ensure treatment access and adherence among those who are less educated, poorer, or less motivated than the patients who have so far come forward also could drive diseconomies. The contribution of these socioeconomic determinants to treatment access and success is not yet well understood.

The Rationing Dilemma: Who Gets a Seat in the Lifeboat?

With the expansion of free treatment beginning to slow, patients needing treatment, their families and friends, health care providers, and patients already benefiting from treatment are becoming acutely aware of the mechanisms that each country and each ART provider adopts to ration care.[28] Whether inadvertently or by government intention, prices increasingly will be used to ration AIDS treatment. As a result, the mix of new patients accepted in ART programs will shift increasingly toward the upper regions of each society's income and wealth distribution. At the lower end of those who can afford treatment, paying for ART will impoverish patients and their families.

It is difficult to estimate the potential impact on poverty in a developing country of any given prevalence of AIDS treatment, but examining the impact of catastrophic health expenditures on household expenditure per capita over a period of one year gives a sense of the problem. I use the case of Bangladesh, even though the data precede the AIDS epidemic, and the country has been largely spared so far. Unfortunately, a similar analysis of catastrophic health expenditures is not yet available for an African country.

Excluding health expenditures, about 20 percent of the Bangladeshi population in 2000 lived in households where daily consumption was less than $1.08 per day, and about 70 percent lived in households below $2.15 per day. But if the traditional measure of household well-being accounts for the health outlays by netting them out, the result is dramatic for some households—indeed, the net consumption per household member for those ostensibly above the poverty line are brought back down below it. Health expenditure large enough to reduce a family to penury can be fairly classified as catastrophic. Even households that would otherwise have been in the top 10 percent of household expenditure were reduced to poverty by one of the two measures once health expenditure was netted out of their annual consumption.[29]

Not all households suffer substantial reductions in well-being from health expenditure. Getting a better grip on prevalence requires another approach, illustrated by table 3-2, which gives the percentage of individuals whose household expenditure net of health care costs is in fact below the poverty line. The table draws on data from four South Asian countries (Van Doorslaer and others 2006).

As table 3-2 shows, in India, this redefinition of poverty would push an additional 20.6 million below the higher poverty line and 37.4 million people below the lower one, increasing the proportion of Indians suffering from the most extreme form of poverty by 12 percent. In Bangladesh, Nepal, and Sri Lanka, health expenditure increases the number of those below the lower poverty line by 17, 6, and 8 percent, respectively.

As the table illustrates, many who seek private-sector treatment for AIDS are likely to be pushed below the poverty line. Suppose that an individual spends approximately $365 per year out of pocket on AIDS treatment, which is enough to cover the full cost of first-line triple-drug therapy at generic prices, plus doctor visits and some laboratory tests. In a four-person household, this would add $0.25 per member to daily health expenditure. Applied to Bangladesh, households at about the fortieth percentile of the country's expenditure distribution, which had no other health expenditure, would be pushed below the lower poverty line by a single AIDS patient, to be on a par with households at the twentieth percentile. Two AIDS patients in a household would severely impoverish a household that had previously been at the forty-fifth percentile of the expenditure distribution.

What would be the result of the impact of out-of-pocket AIDS treatment expenditure on poverty in India? Suppose that the distributions of overall expenditure and health expenditure for the poorest 40 percent of India's population are similar to those of the lowest 40 percent of the Bangladeshi population. Further suppose that all the 500,000–1,600,000 people who are estimated to be living with AIDS in India are in households that would otherwise be above the $1.08 poverty line but not above the fortieth percentile of the Indian income distribution. Because between 300 million and 500 million Indians were living under the $1.08 poverty line in 2000, AIDS would increase the number of strictly poor by less than 0.5 percent. In so doing, it would increase the percentage of the population below the stricter poverty line by about 3 percent, from about 35 percent to 38 percent. Thus, in any single year the expenditures on AIDS treatment might increase India's number of poor by about 10 percent.

The impact might be worse if we were able to account for the fact that AIDS treatment must continue for the rest of the patient's life—in other words, it is more like a chronic illness than an acute illness. A household might recover its economic status after a single catastrophic expenditure depresses net expenditure for a single year. But that same household would need more robust coping strategies to deal with a stream of catastrophic expenditures over several years. To analyze chronic disease, one would need to look at wealth (or permanent income) instead of expenditure. To push

TABLE 3-2. Population below the Poverty Line in South Asia before and after Paying Out-of-Pocket Health Expenses

| | Poverty line of $1.08 per day/change in poverty head count | | | | | Poverty line of $2.15 per day/change in poverty head count | | | | |
| | Percent below poverty line | | | | | Percent below poverty line | | | | |
Country	Pre-payment	Post-payment	Percentage point change	Number of individuals	Percent change	Pre-payment	Post-payment	Percentage point change	Number of individuals	Percent change
Bangladesh	22.5	26.3	3.8	4,940,585	16.8	73.0	76.5	3.5	4,653,875	4.9
India	31.1	34.8	3.7	37,358,760	11.9	80.3	82.4	2.1	20,638,361	2.6
Kenya	19.7	...	...	n.a.	...	39.9	...	...	n.a.	...
Nepal	39.3	41.6	2.2	515,933	5.7	80.4	81.7	1.3	290,280	1.6
Sri Lanka	3.8	4.1	0.3	60,116	8.3	39.1	40.8	1.7	325,783	4.3
Uganda	51.5	...	...	n.a.	...	75.6	...	...	n.a.	...

Source: Van Doorslaer, Wagstaff, and Rutten 1993; Van Doorslaer and others 2006, 2007; Over 2009a.
n.a. = not available.

this analysis further, it also would be necessary to have information on the distribution of HIV infections across the income or expenditure distributions for the most severely affected countries in Africa and Asia, as well as the poverty and health expenditure data depicted in table 3-2. While a poverty head count can be estimated for any country with a household expenditure survey, until recently no population-based information has been available on the distribution of HIV infection by socioeconomic class in almost any country in the world.[30]

Using these new data, it will be possible to predict the impact of any given rate of uptake of free ART and any ART-rationing rule on poverty. Such calculations drive home the equity issues that out-of-pocket expenditures for AIDS treatment raise and may enable estimates of the impact on out-of-pocket ART expenditure and poverty of any public-sector decision regarding the uptake of patients on publicly financed ART. Besides delineating the social impact of any rationing decision, this type of analysis highlights the importance of preventing HIV, especially among poor people, who can least afford to pay.

Indirect Effects of AIDS Treatment

Recognizing the direct benefits of AIDS treatment funding for the millions of people whose lives it prolongs, this chapter focuses primarily on the fiscal and dependency burdens these entitlements engender and strategies to mitigate them. But the story of the impact of AIDS treatment would be incomplete without a discussion of the possible indirect effects of its expansion, both beneficial and perverse. To the extent that these indirect effects are beneficial, they alleviate some of the pressure for mitigation. To the extent they are perverse, recognizing their threat can forewarn policymakers to avoid them and work even more urgently toward the AIDS transition.

Possible Macroeconomic Benefits of AIDS Treatment

Public-sector support of ART for AIDS patients could benefit the economy as a whole for several reasons. To the extent that ART extends the productive life of AIDS patients, it enables households, communities, and employers to receive greater returns on previous investments in the patients' education and on the job training. This effect has the potential not only to improve productivity, but also to encourage private investment in human capital.

In addition, publicly financed AIDS treatment constitutes a fiscal stimulus that—given sufficient flexibility in the supply of domestic inputs such as health personnel—can expand employment and stimulate economic growth. In severely affected countries where AIDS treatment is extended to a large fraction of the adult population, this stimulus and the consequent multiplier effect on growth could be substantial.

Government-sponsored ART also removes a potential obstacle to foreign direct investment that generates employment, acting as a kind of employment subsidy. In comparison to an alternative in which the government asked foreign and domestic investors to subsidize ART for all their employees in need, a publicly financed ART program could stimulate foreign investment and thus boost economic growth.

Finally, if the alternative to public-sector financing of ART delivery is private financing and delivery of ART with much lower adherence rates, public-sector ART financing may be preventing or slowing the domestic and international spread of drug-resistant strains of HIV. Although only applicable if public-sector ART financing ensures high adherence, this consideration could be the most important for the longer-run welfare of individual countries and for global public health.[31] While these benefits are hypothetically substantial in a severely affected country, they can only be attained to the degree that AIDS treatment itself can be financed from public and private sources. Planning explicitly for an AIDS transition will help government and donors commit to such long-term financing.

Effects of AIDS Treatment on Other Health Care

A long-time source of heated debate has been whether AIDS treatment helps or hurts health systems—a topic on which the empirical data are sparse. Some anecdotal reports suggest AIDS treatment can create a two-tiered health system, with resources drawn out of the second, "lower" tier of general primary and secondary care into the "upper" tier of AIDS treatment. But before-and-after photographs from Rwanda, for example, show the dramatic improvement in the physical condition of a health center after it has been remodeled with AIDS treatment money. A major problem in addressing the effect of AIDS treatment on these health care facilities is to know what would have happened in them if AIDS treatment had not been introduced (Price and others 2007). In other words, in the absence of PEPFAR, would the Rwandan health centers have been strengthened anyway by donor money? And are the instances of strengthening in Rwanda and elsewhere only temporary, to be followed by decay? Indeed, the before-and-after photographs of a Rwandan health center could plausibly be reversed to tell the story of how past health center improvements have been followed by lack of maintenance and then decay. So with these experiences of past refurbishments followed by decay, the question is whether the apparent health system improvements accompanying current AIDS treatment financing will be any more sustainable.

The good news is that this whole debate is fast becoming moot. In 2009 the Obama administration announced the Global Health Initiative, which integrates the PEPFAR program within efforts to strengthen developing-country health systems more generally. In the future, AIDS programs will be judged at least in part by their contributions to health system functioning. The challenge will be how to measure whether the health systems are indeed becoming stronger.

Effects of AIDS Treatment on HIV Prevention: Good and Bad

If a person suffering from an infectious disease like tuberculosis or syphilis is cured of that disease, the individual can no longer infect others. Thus, in these cases the treatment improves the population's health not only by helping the treated patient, but also by preventing that patient from infecting others. Whether ART for AIDS helps slow the spread of the infection is not so clear. As briefly discussed in chapter 1 and illustrated with table 1-1, ART has biological and behavioral effects on HIV prevention—some of which are potentially beneficial, slowing the spread of the epidemic, and others that are potentially harmful, speeding its spread.

TREATMENT REDUCES INFECTIOUSNESS. Effective AIDS treatment reduces the number of virus cells in the blood stream to undetectable levels. Biological studies show that patients who are effectively adhering to ART are less likely to transmit infection during unprotected sex than they would be if they remained untreated during the last year of life. In addition, a study on ART patients in Côte d'Ivoire who were counseled to maintain safe behavior showed no increase in self-reported risk behavior (Katzenstein, Laga, and Moatti 2003). A recent study in Rwanda finds the same encouraging result using biological markers for unprotected sex (Dunkle and others 2008).

The question is whether this beneficial "externality" for the sexual partner of an AIDS patient is sufficiently strong and generalizable to justify greatly expanded ART on prevention grounds. Recent discussion has centered on the so-called test-and-treat strategy of annually testing the entire population and beginning treatment immediately for those who test positive. Randomized controlled trials are under way in Washington, D.C., and the Bronx, New York, that should yield more information on the efficacy of this approach. Unfortunately, as explained by the analysis in the second chapter, a test-and-treat strategy would cost between two-and-a-half and four times the cost of recent expansion policies, from which donors are already pulling back. Also as described in chapter 2, epidemiological models find that a plausibly operational version of this strategy could not control the epidemic without considerable behavioral change toward safer sexual or drug-injecting behavior.

TREATMENT STIMULATES THE DEMAND FOR TESTING. Treatment availability unquestionably stimulates the demand for HIV testing, which in turn stimulates the demand for AIDS treatment among those who find themselves to be HIV-positive. This seemingly virtuous circle ensures that those with unmet need for treatment increasingly will express a political demand and, for those with purchasing power, an economic demand for treatment. This is one of the important dynamics of AIDS treatment that increases the pressure for higher spending. Unfortunately, as discussed in chapter 2, HIV testing does not necessarily lead to reduced risk behavior. For this behavioral effect of treatment to strongly reinforce HIV prevention, other measures will be required. Perhaps by channeling the increased demand for testing into couples testing, this effect would become unambiguously beneficial for prevention.

TREATMENT MAY INHIBIT OR DISINHIBIT RISK BEHAVIOR. Data from antenatal clinics in some African countries show that after years of public health messages on the dangers of risky sex, the prevalence of HIV has declined among young women (Ghys and others 2010). Since these data cover years prior to the wide availability of ART, it suggests that at least in some African populations, fear of AIDS and knowledge of which behaviors are risky have inhibited risk behavior. Now that treatment is increasingly available, the question is whether and how expanded free access to HIV treatment affects the risk behavior of those who are sexually active or use injection drugs.

One possibility is that expanded treatment access inhibits the risk behavior not only of those on treatment but also of the general population, perhaps by reducing the stigma associated with HIV prevention as well as treatment. While the test-and-treat strategy discussed above and in chapter 2 depends primarily on a biological effect of treatment to reduce the infectivity of the treated individual, the original proponents of that strategy also argued that universal treatment availability would have such a beneficial effect on risk behavior (Granich and others 2009).

Unfortunately, few studies have examined the impact of expanded treatment access on risk behavior of the much larger population of adults not yet on treatment or not even infected. In one recent study in Mozambique, where AIDS treatment has been rapidly expanding, Damien de Walque,

Oklahoma State professor Harounan Kazianga, and I found evidence that the false belief that AIDS can be cured, perhaps engendered by improved access to AIDS treatment, seemed to increase men's demand for risky sexual behavior (de Walque, Kazianga, and Over 2010).

Other than reducing their risk behavior, as some studies suggest might have happened, Africans may have attempted to protect themselves against AIDS by marrying earlier. Given that the trend away from extremely early marriage by African girls has been heralded as a mark of socioeconomic development with important benefits for children, it would be unfortunate if young women were responding to the AIDS threat by seeking safe haven in earlier marriage (Case 2009). This would be especially problematic if, as some contend, marriage were to increase the risk of HIV infection. Thus, a previously unnoticed benefit of effective treatment could be to reassure young women that they can remain single longer and thereby encourage a healthy postponement of marriage into the twenties.

TREATMENT INCREASES EXPOSURE TO AN INFECTED PERSON. Because ART typically prolongs the healthy life of an HIV-infected person by many years but does not cure AIDS, that person has more opportunity to infect others. This biological effect of ART on exposure is more worrisome if the patient is not adhering perfectly to the medication and therefore not suppressing viral replication.

TREATMENT CAN SELECT FOR RESISTANT STRAINS OF HIV. In 2010 the WHO reported that 5–15 percent of a sample of fifty-two consecutively diagnosed HIV-positive women in Ouagadougou, Burkina Faso, were found to be carrying a drug-resistant strain (WHO, UNAIDS, and UNICEF 2010, 65). Since these women were between 15 and 24 years old, pregnant for the first time, and not yet on ART, they probably had contracted a drug-resistant strain of HIV from a sexual partner. Because treating their strains of HIV requires immediate access to costly, harder-to-find, harder-to-manage second-line therapy, they will have a harder time initiating and adhering to treatment. If treatment had never been available in their community, any HIV they would have contracted would have been easier to treat. So the fact that treatment selects for resistant strains of HIV is a negative biological effect of treatment on prevention.

Ensuring HIV Prevention through Better Treatment

In an ideal world, the accelerated expansion of access to AIDS treatment would somehow slow AIDS transmission, automatically extinguishing the epidemic. In such a world, there would be no tension between the immediate, palpable objective of treating sick people and the far-sighted, abstract objective of preventing HIV infections. The AIDS transition could be accomplished by investing solely in treatment expansion and allowing its beneficial effects on HIV prevention to work their magic. However, in the real world, the beneficial spillover effects of AIDS treatment on HIV prevention are offset by perverse spillovers and thus on balance do not appear to be sufficient to bring the annual number of new infections down below the annual death rate. In the absence of much more effective prevention, successful treatment expansion will indefinitely augment the number of people with AIDS treatment entitlements, forever postponing the date of an AIDS transition.

In chapter 2, I present some specific ideas for improving HIV prevention by the application of incentives. In this chapter, I present ideas for applying incentives in the domain of AIDS treatment, not only to improve its effectiveness, but also to strengthen the beneficial effects of AIDS treatment on HIV prevention. If we can design reward systems for AIDS treatment programs that align the incentives of all who benefit from them more perfectly with the interests of the governments and donors who are funding the AIDS programs, we will have pushed this world a little closer to a place where AIDS treatment unequivocally reduces new infections in the general population, thereby reducing future demands on the public purse and contributing to reducing its own burden.

Performance-Based Funding for AIDS Treatment

A relatively new policy instrument for the health sector is the application of performance-based incentives (PBIs) to increase the productivity or improve the quality of health care. These incentives are defined as "the transfer of money or material goods conditional on taking a measurable action or achieving a predetermined performance target." They include "incentives on both the demand and the supply sides, at both individual and collective levels, [which operate at] the interface between provider and patient." But they exclude "the conditional payments that donor agencies offer to national [or sub-national] governments" (Eichler, Levine, and Performance-Based Incentives Working Group 2009, 6).[32] Typical PBIs include conditional cash transfers, transportation subsidies, food support, and financial rewards to providers for results (or penalties for poor performance).

One country that has experimented with PBIs for health care delivery for many years is Rwanda (Eichler, Levine, and Performance-Based Incentives Working Group 2009, 189–214). In 2006, when it began to scale up PBIs to its entire health care delivery system, Rwanda decided to permit rigorous evaluation of the PBI approach, which had been under way since 2002. To do so, the government allocated PBI rewards to 79 of 165 facilities and withheld the reward system from 86 facilities. The assignment was partly random and partly based on matching criteria, so that the facilities with PBI would be as similar as possible to those without it. During the period from 2006 to 2008, Rwanda also was scaling up AIDS treatment in the same facilities. To ensure that the provision of this additional complex service did not confound the evaluation, Rwanda balanced the AIDS treatment rollout between the groups with PBI rewards and those without.

How did the PBIs work? Preliminary results show that health personnel exposed to the PBIs were more productive than personnel who were not (Gertler and others 2009). Furthermore, the health personnel with better training and knowledge responded more to the incentives. These results held for all facilities, including those with integrated HIV/AIDS diagnosis and treatment services. Even so, the results suggest that while the mere presence of AIDS services actually increased child preventive care, the presence of AIDS services combined with a PBI system more than offset this beneficial effect. Thus, care must be taken to adjust the relative strength of the incentives across different types of services if the intention is not to reduce other services.

In addition, other studies show that PBI systems can improve patient return for test results (Chaisson and others 1996; Thornton 2008) and improve patient adherence to ART—for example, by providing transportation vouchers (Sorensen and others 2007). By deploying these types of PBI systems, governments can hope to outsource critical HIV-prevention and treatment services to the private sector.

Yet another type of PBI aimed at improving incentives for successful AIDS treatment would be to outsource the monitoring of providers to patients. Such a system could substitute for, and perhaps improve on, a portion of the expensive and logistically challenging monitoring that a central authority would otherwise perform. Treatment resources would be allocated to accredited groups of ART patients instead of to health care providers or facilities.[33] Patient groups would receive training in advocacy and be charged with ensuring the precise adherence of each group member, whose CD4 counts would be monitored. Those groups in a given geographic region that succeed in sustaining and improving the clinical indicators for existing members would be the first to receive the allocation of a new treatment slot when one is available. Furthermore, a given group of patients also would be able to move its treatment budget from one group of providers to another. By giving the group of ART clients more bargaining power vis-à-vis the health care providers than any one of them would have alone, such an approach would inject into the subsidized transaction between patient and health care provider an element of market discipline and accountability.

The idea of expanding patient groups that are more successful can reach beyond treatment to influence the rate of HIV transmission in the general population. Suppose that the allocation of new treatment slots to patient groups were conditioned not only on how well they sustain the adherence of their members, but also on how well they contribute to reduced HIV incidence in a selected nearby community. For example, suppose a patient support group is composed of former prostitutes who had worked in the same risky neighborhood context. Such a group could designate that same neighborhood as their HIV-prevention target, and they could be judged on their outreach activities to prostitutes who work there and their clients. While measurement of prevention effectiveness would be challenging for the government or donor authorized to allocate the incremental treatment slots, the groups could compete with one another on how to demonstrate their prevention effectiveness.

While based on a competitive model, such an arrangement would intentionally mute the competitive pressures to avoid several possible unintended consequences. For example, in a truly competitive model, unsuccessful firms go out of business. In this context, the dissolution of a patient support group might leave patients without support, endangering their lives. Therefore, I propose that the competition only be for incremental slots, not for existing ones.

Another unintended consequence of excessive competition might be hostility between competing patient support groups. Qualitative work by anthropologists and ethnologists to design an appropriate reward structure can mitigate this risk. For example, in many cultural contexts a winner-take-all reward structure that gives all new incremental treatment slots to the single best–performing patient support group might turn friendly competition into adversarial conflict. One way to reduce this risk is to lower the stakes of the competition by distributing available slots to several groups, in proportion to their performance scores.

To avoid either of these unintended consequences, additional incremental treatment slots must be available each year. This approach to create incentive-compatible reward structures, leveraging treatment demand for the benefit of prevention, can only work if donors and governments continue to expand treatment rolls at substantial uptake rates.

Cash on Delivery for AIDS Treatment

Over and above the PBI mechanisms for patients and providers, a cash-on-delivery (COD) system could improve treatment outcomes and exert additional leverage on prevention. As discussed in chapter 2, COD applies incentives to the top levels of governmental organization—such as the state, the province, or the nation—in recognition that top-level leadership on the issue of HIV/AIDS is critical.[34] The COD approach aims to help donors facilitate longer-term commitments to sustained effort on a particular objective by establishing a reward mechanism that provides payments for the achievement of specific objectives, payments that governments can use to motivate actors and their constituencies at every level. It is quite explicitly a reward or a prize that the country or state has won because of its achievement of a challenging, worthwhile, internationally recognized social objective. For example, Center for Global Development president Nancy Birdsall, writing first with colleagues Owen Barder (2006) and William Savedoff (2010), suggests that a payment of $100 per child be made to the recipient government for every additional child who completes primary school.

Application of the COD approach to the provision of ART for AIDS patients has much in common with its application to education. In both cases, a COD program contract would need to recognize and reward "enrollment" and "persistence" in the program. The education concept of enrollment can be compared to the medical concept of treatment initiation; regular attendance to primary school completion is analogous to successful long-term adherence to medication. A COD program for AIDS treatment thus would reward a government for improvements in the total number of patients to have successfully adhered to treatment for a specified length of time, according to a payout rule agreed to in advance.

Furthermore, in both education and AIDS treatment, enrollment is much more valuable to an individual if it occurs at the appropriate time in that person's life. The student who waits too long to start school loses forever the opportunity to maximize the benefits of schooling. Similarly an AIDS patient who waits too long to start treatment has a worse prognosis than a patient who begins treatment promptly on attaining ART eligibility. Thus an appropriate payout rule should reward timely initiation of treatment, without excessively penalizing unavoidably tardy initiation. Given these structural similarities between primary education and AIDS treatment, lessons learned in either of these areas might be applicable to the other. Transferable lessons might include the nature of a feasible reward structure and the best systems for auditing results.

The COD approach to funding AIDS treatment has several advantages as a supplement to current funding approaches. First, with a properly structured reward or payout rule, COD can reward all dimensions of treatment success, not just the total number enrolled in treatment. A treatment program that accepts many people but fails to sustain each one is unacceptable.[35] This imbalance can be addressed by designing the payout rule so that it rewards a patient's survival for an additional month at a higher rate than it rewards a month of treatment for a new patient. By rewarding a treatment program for the survival of its patients, the COD system will automatically reward adherence, quality of care, and early recruitment. By also rewarding the total number enrolled in treatment, the COD system will encourage an AIDS treatment program to reach out to ever-larger numbers, including poor people.

When a COD system is first appended to a traditional command-driven system based on reimbursement of full costs plus overheads, its incremental effect hopefully will be to encourage the recipients and their partners to produce more and better treatment with the same resources— that is, to become more efficient. If the donors decide to gradually shift the mix of resources so that a larger fraction over time is paid in the COD component and a smaller share as cost-plus reimbursement for inputs, the COD's power to improve efficiency would increase.

One essential ingredient for the success of a COD program for AIDS treatment will be establishing, at the time the COD agreement is signed, a mutually agreeable method for measuring the results against which the program will pay rewards. Donors and recipients must agree not only on which results to reward but also on how to measure those results, who will do the measurement, and who will audit them. The difficulty of this measurement problem is directly related to the number of patients under treatment.

For example, out of 125 low- and middle-income countries receiving donor funding for AIDS treatment, 57 need to keep track of fewer than 5,000 patients—a much more manageable task than keeping track of all the students who would be the subject of a COD education program in any country. Another 50 countries currently treat, or need to treat, between 10,000 and 60,000 patients. These countries will find measurement more challenging, but with assistance in the construction and maintenance of a strong patient data management system, they should be able to provide results data on all their patients. Only for the twenty or thirty countries with treatment rolls exceeding 60,000 patients and those with the weakest patient data management systems might it be necessary to use a representative survey of patients rather than complete data on all of them.

Just as PBI systems at the level of the provider or patient-support group can measure and reward prevention as well as treatment, a COD system also can integrate the rewards for both essential components of any AIDS control program. A comprehensive COD contract for a given country should propose a top-level payout system for both HIV prevention and AIDS treatment that also encourages national, sectoral, and sub-national decisionmakers to reward both dimensions of AIDS program success. That way, chances are greater that lower-level social entrepreneurs will invent mechanisms we have not yet thought of for aligning the interests of providers, patients, and risk-takers more closely with one another and with the country at large in the interests of sustaining AIDS mortality reductions and achieving the AIDS transition.

After seven years of enhanced effort on AIDS treatment, the international community has achieved much, but the AIDS treatment challenge only seems to be growing. By adopting the goal of the AIDS transition, the community of donors and recipients can ensure that treatment uptake continues and contributes in measureable ways to slowing HIV transmission. Joint success in these efforts in turn will open up fiscal space to continue treatment for decades to come.

Alternative Approaches to Estimating the Average Cost of Antiretroviral Treatment

While there have been many studies of the cost of HIV-prevention activities, the cross-country determinants of the cost of antiretroviral therapy (ART) have not yet been estimated.[1] In theory, one would expect that average costs in a country would increase with its level of wealth and decrease with the number of patients it treats (due to economies of scale). Beyond these two factors, one would hope that the individual facilities providing ART services and the country at large would improve efficiency over time. It also might be the case that the availability of donor support for ART would reduce incentives to economize and therefore inflate costs.

In the absence of a cross-country sample of facility cost data, I look for the influence of these potential determinants of cost by analyzing the expenditures on ART that individual countries reported to UNAIDS, the Joint United Nations Program on HIV/AIDS, as part of their UNGASS-mandated reporting requirements.[2] Figure A-1 demonstrates that a country's national income and the total number of patients treated do indeed explain about a third of observed variation in average costs. A country whose per capita income is 10 percent higher will spend on average about 8.5 percent more per patient-year. For example, the average expenditure per patient in 2007 of a country with 25,000 patients under treatment would be $296 dollars if the country's per capita income were $460, $835 if the country's per capita income were $2,000, and $1,690 if the country's per capita income were $5,430.[3]

123

FIGURE A-1. Average Costs of Antiretroviral Therapy (ART) Rise with National Income and Fall with Number of ART Patients

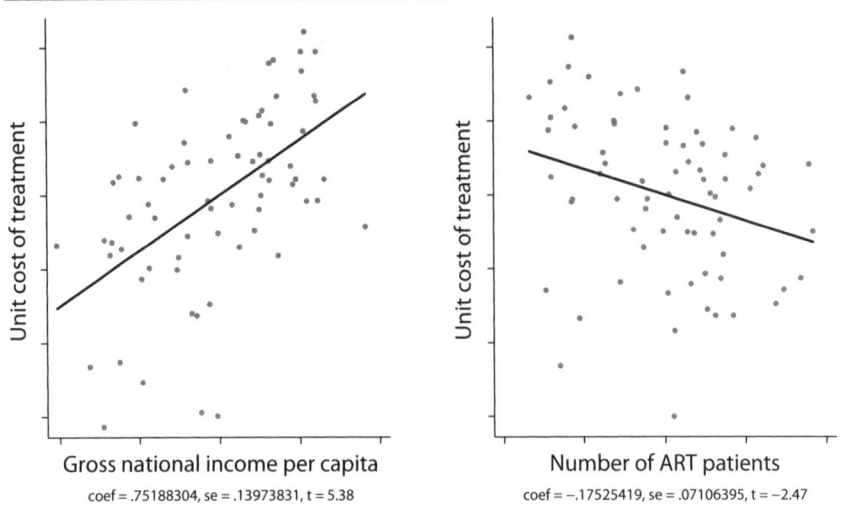

Gross national income per capita
coef = .75188304, se = .13973831, t = 5.38

Number of ART patients
coef = −.17525419, se = .07106395, t = −2.47

Source: Author's calculations based on data from Annex 2 of UNAIDS 2008.
Note: These scatter plots display the partial effects of gross national income per capita and of total ART patients, holding constant the other variable and a dummy variable for the year. Each axis measures the residuals from the regression of the given variable on the omitted variable. The plots were created with Stata 11's avplot command.

The number of enrolled patients also affects the cost. Based on the regression results illustrated in Figure A-1, Figure A-2 shows how the number of enrolled patients reduces the predicted level of total ART expenditure per enrolled patient for countries at three different income levels. A country with a 10 percent larger patient enrollment benefits from about a 1.5 percent reduction in average cost per patient. Thus, an upper-middle-income country with an income per capita of $5,430 would spend $1,690 per patient-year when treating 25,000 patients, but only about $1,500 per patient-year if it doubles its treatment rolls to 50,000 patients.

Other factors besides per capita income and number of enrolled patients have influenced the 86 percent drop in costs in nominal terms between 2005 and 2007. Given that the drug component decreased by only about 50 percent, the rest of the reduction must have occurred either in the quantity of health services used per patient or in the average fixed cost per patient. The most likely explanation is that 2005 saw large investments in capacity without commensurate increases in the number of patients, which then occurred the following two years.

Pulling all these data together, I project future costs of treatment. First, I assume that reductions from lower drug prices and lower average fixed

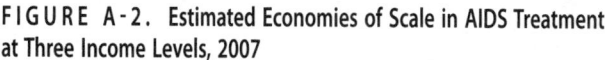

FIGURE A-2. Estimated Economies of Scale in AIDS Treatment
at Three Income Levels, 2007

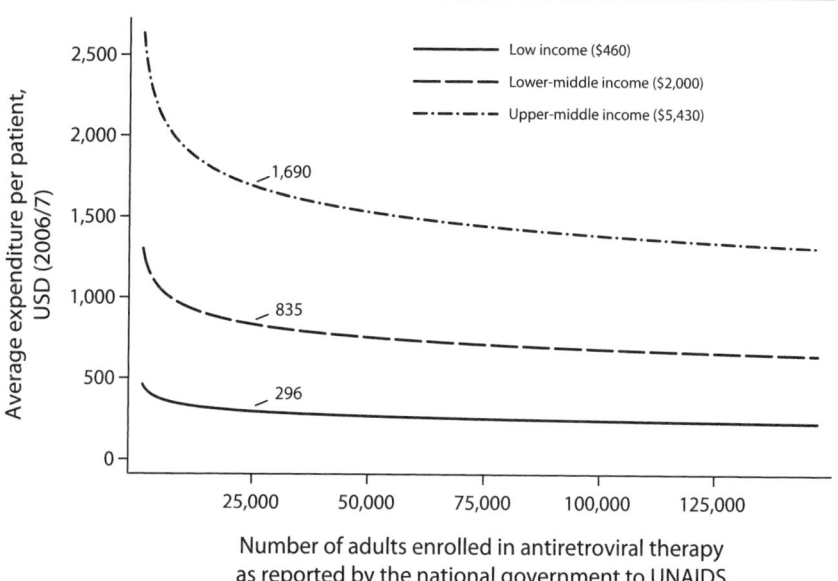

Source: Author's calculations.

costs have stabilized,[4] but I allow future average cost reductions owing to economies of scale from the increased numbers of enrolled patients.[5] Conversely, if countries shrink their treatment programs—either because of successful prevention or fiscal constraints—the average cost per treated patient will rise by about 1.5 percent for every 10 percent reduction in treatment numbers.

Second, I assume a pronounced positive correlation between a country's income per capita and all components of the unit cost of delivering ART. Indeed, countries with higher incomes have paid as much as double the cost that lower-income countries have paid for exactly the same drugs. The income elasticity of per patient expenditure on ART is about 0.71 so that a country with 10 percent higher income per capita will spend about 7 percent more per patient. This suggests that future income growth will drive future growth in per-patient AIDS treatment expenditure, though not at the same rate.

The result of these calculations is that the average cost for AIDS treatment will remain relatively stable.

A Meta-Analysis of the Health Benefits of Early Initiation of Antiretroviral Therapy

This appendix presents my methods for estimating the benefits of earlier recruitment to antiretroviral therapy (ART). I base my approach on a systematic comparison of published data on the survival of patients who start treatment in the early stages of infection and those who start late. Figure B-1 shows that without treatment, an HIV-infected person has a probability of death approaching certainty as the CD4 count approaches zero. However, treatment reduces mortality dramatically for those who are able to adhere to the treatment regime and are retained by the treatment program. For those who start treatment when their CD4 count is 400 or above, estimated first-year mortality is about 0.04 (about 4 percent). This percentage rises to 10 percent for a starting CD4 count of 50 and then rapidly rises toward 100 percent as the CD4 level approaches zero. Moreover, every 10 percent decline in CD4 at ART initiation is associated with a 4 percent rise in first-year mortality.[6]

Unfortunately, this approach to estimating the benefits of earlier ART initiation is subject to at least two sources of bias. First, the estimates leave out the mortality of those who dropped out of treatment programs and could not be traced; mortality for these patients is likely to be higher than for those who continued treatment. Researchers who have attempted to trace those who have stopped attending their treatment sessions have learned the fate of fewer than half of them. One recent review of these studies found that about 40 percent of the former patients who were suc-

FIGURE B-1. Expected First-Year Mortality Depends on CD4 Count at Treatment Initiation

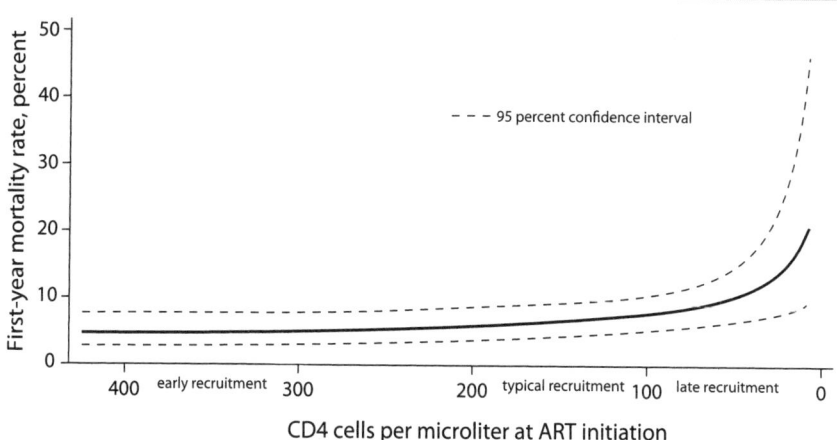

CD4 cells per microliter at ART initiation

Note: assumes that mortality rate for those lost to follow-up is 0 percent.

Source: Author's calculations based on Fox, McCarthy and Over (2011).

cessfully traced had died within the year, and it seems likely that the mortality rate among the untraced was even higher (Brinkhof, Pujades-Rodriguez, and Egger 2009). This omission is likely to underestimate the mortality of those on ART, especially at low CD4 counts. Second, the data might exclude the mortality of those with less severe symptoms at any stage in their disease because they did not seek care—an omission that is likely to overestimate the mortality of those on ART, especially at high CD4 counts.

I attempt to correct for these two biases in three steps. First, I estimate the mortality of the patients who are lost to follow up and use it to adjust upward the curve in figure B-1. The curve labeled "meta-analysis of mortality on ART" in figure B-2 shows that this adjustment estimates a substantially higher first-year mortality of patients starting ART than would be apparent from the retained patients alone.[7]

Second, I use the latest estimates from historical cohorts who did not have access to treatment to anchor mortality at the highest CD4 counts (eART-linc 2008). Figure B-2 shows this by overlaying the adjusted mortality estimates of those on ART on the relationship between mortality and CD4 count at initiation for those not on ART, derived from the historical cohorts (eART-linc 2008). The intersection of the two lines at a CD4 count

FIGURE B-2. Mortality during the Forthcoming Year by CD4 Count

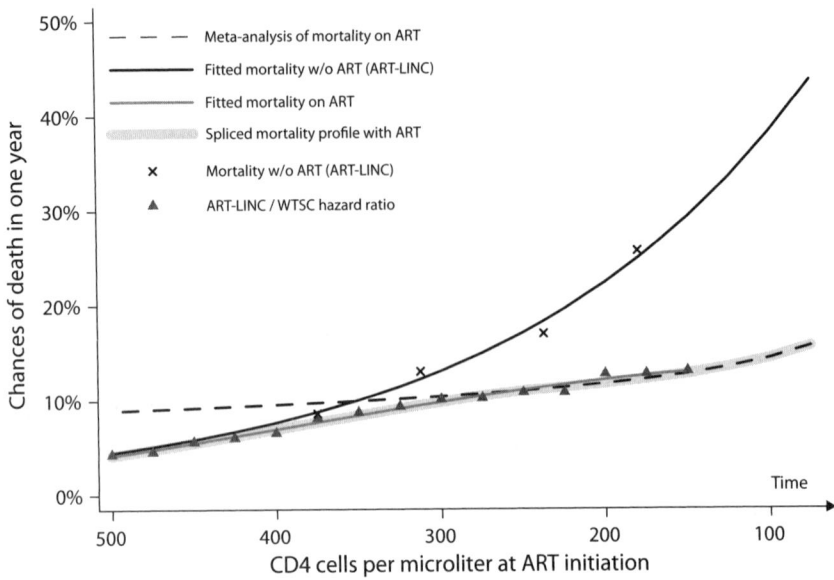

Source: Author's construction from figure B-2, using data from eART-linc 2008, When to Start Consortium, and Sterne 2009, and results from Fox, McCarthy, and Over 2011.

Note: The AIDSCost model assumes that mortality among those who begin treatment at a given CD4 is the smaller of two mortality rates: (a) the author's meta-analysis of the first-year mortality on antiretroviral therapy (ART) by CD4 count at ART initiation and (b) the rate from the ART-linc study on mortality by CD4 count among those not on ART. The solid triangles show that comparing the mortality risk between the ART-linc data and the When to Start Consortium data (WTSC) to produce a hazard ratio yields an incremental mortality risk roughly equal to that obtained from the spliced relationship.

of about 350 is implausible because it would imply that starting ART at a CD4 count above 350 would increase the patient's risk of death compared to not starting treatment at all. Instead, one can interpret this intersection as confirmation that the existing estimates of ART-patient mortality are unrealistically high for patients who started with high CD4 counts.

Third, I use the latest high-income country estimates of the hazard from incrementally postponing ART to splice together the two estimates from low-income countries. One approach to estimating the benefits of ART by the CD4 count at which patients are enrolled is to reconcile the two sources of information by assuming there are no treatment benefits above a CD4 count of 350. In this case, one would assume that first-year mortality on ART is the minimum of the two curves in figure B-2. However, this hypothesis is inconsistent with the latest information from high-income countries on the benefits of early initiation (When to Start Consortium and Sterne 2009). An approach that recognizes the potential mortality reduction even in low-income countries of earlier treatment initiation uses these estimates of the incremental hazard from ART postponement in high-income countries to infer the reduced mortality risk at high CD4 counts—while relying on the meta-analysis for estimates of mortality at low CD4 counts. Figure B-2 illustrates this approach.[8] I derive the health benefits of ART that are estimated in this book for different CD4 initiation thresholds from the difference between estimated no-ART mortality shown in Figure B-2 as the line labeled "fitted mortality w/o ART" and the estimated mortality on ART shown in the figure as the line labeled "spliced mortality profile with ART."

A Model for Projecting Future AIDS Treatment Costs

AIDSCost, the model I use to project the costs of AIDS treatment in this book, includes a compartment-based difference equation of the spread of the epidemic and a simple model of the unit cost of treating a patient. The AIDSCost model is available for download from www.cgdev.org/aidscost, and the code is open source.[9] Because the model runs using the Stata statistical software, a copy of that program is necessary to execute the model.[10]

To use AIDSCost, one can select values of any parameters listed in table C-1 or leave the parameters unspecified to run the model with the default values listed in the table. The uptake parameter is the only one that does not have a default value; instead, it specifies the user's assumption regarding the proportion of unmet need for treatment that will be added to treatment rolls each year in each country. The user may select any individual value between zero and one, and the value is then used to model uptake in every country in the simulation. Alternatively, the user can direct the program to use the idiosyncratic, country-specific uptake rates that are embodied in the cross-country data available with the program.

For most of the projections in the book, I eschew making the many assumptions required to model HIV incidence in favor of the assumption that absolute incidence—that is, the absolute number of new cases per year—declines at a constant user-specified rate. Annual rates of decrease in figure 1-5, for example, include 0 percent, 3 percent, and 10 percent. This

TABLE C-1. Parameters Used in the AIDS Cost Program

	Name	Default value
Patient recruitment		
Scale-up of first-line treatment modeled as constant proportion, sigma,		
of unmet need, where sigma is constant across all countries and equal to:	sigma	User defined
The median CD4 count at antiretroviral therapy (ART) initiation	cd4	130
Proportion of HIV-positive newly eligible for ART	erate	0.111
Incidence is modeled as endogenous to ART and affected by prevention scale-up		
Incidence rate in core group, year 0	ir0	.2
Maximum HIV prevention effort	maxep	.6
Start year of circumcision and effort	pstrtyr	2010
Target year of maximum circumcision and effort	ptrgtyr	2025
Circumcision		
Maximum proportion circumcised	maxcp	.8
Protection of circumcision: csp = 1 is perfect	csp	.6
Vaccination		
Maximum proportion vaccinated	maxvp	.7
Protection of vaccine: ve=1 perfect	ve	.6
Start year of vaccination scale-up	vstrtyr	2025
Target year of maximum vaccination scale-up	vtrgtyr	2040
Treatment effects		
Fraction transmission after primary infection	fp	.7
Protection of treatment: gp = 1 perfect	gp	.8
Max disinhibition of ART on treated < 1	maxdt	0
Max disinhibition of ART on untreated < inf	maxdu	0

(continued)

range spans all declines in the number of new infections that most observers would find plausible and thus permits me to project a date of a future AIDS transition using relatively few parameters and assumptions.

The most recent version of AIDSCost available on the Center for Global Development website allows the user an alternative, assumption-rich approach to projecting future incidence. Figure C-1 presents the parameter-entry dialog available to the user for modeling the impact of four classes of policy on new cases: male circumcision, vaccination, antiretroviral treatment, and a catch-all category called "effort." This parameterization of the model, currently in version 4.05, results from a collaborative effort between Geoffrey Garnett of Imperial College and me.

TABLE C-1. Parameters Used in the AIDS Cost Program *(continued)*

	Name	Default value
Projection period		
First year of projections (projection take-off)	takeoff	2010
Last year of projections (projection horizon)	horizon	2020
Second-line treatment		
Second-line ART to start in year	strtyr	2009
Second-line ART to reach target in year	trgtyr	2020
Starting coverage rate for second-line ART[a]	strtcov2	Region specific
Target coverage rate for second-line ART	trgtcov2	0.95
Mortality		
Death rate of patients during their first year on first-line ART	adrate1	0.133
Death rate during subsequent years on first-line ART	adrate2	0.04
Death rate of patients on second-line ART	bdrate	0.04
Death rate of patients who are eligible for ART but are not enrolled in ART	ndrate	0.325
Cost computations based on following parameters:		
Lower bound for first-line drug costs[b]	rxc1lb	$88
Upper bound for first-line drug costs	rxc1ub	$261
Lower bound for second-line drug costs	rxc2lb	$819
Upper bound for second-line drug costs	rxc2ub	$2,634
Number of bed-days per year per patient	hsbedn	1.56
Number of outpatient visits per patient	hsvstn	9.5
Average fixed non-drug cost at ART=1000	nonrxcaf	$750
Elasticity of average fixed cost of ART with respect to the number of ART patients	scale	−0.142

Note: The parameter definitions and their default values in this table apply to AIDSCost Version 4.x.

a. The model embodies the assumption that for those people who fail first-line ART, access to second-line ART expands linearly from about 5 percent of all patients needing it now to 95 percent of all patients needing it in 2020.

b. Drug costs are assumed to vary across countries with the 2007 GDP per capita of the country according to the patterns observed by the World Health Organization in 2006 and then remain constant in any given country over time.

FIGURE C-1. Incidence Modeling Tab, Version 4.05 of the AIDSCost Program

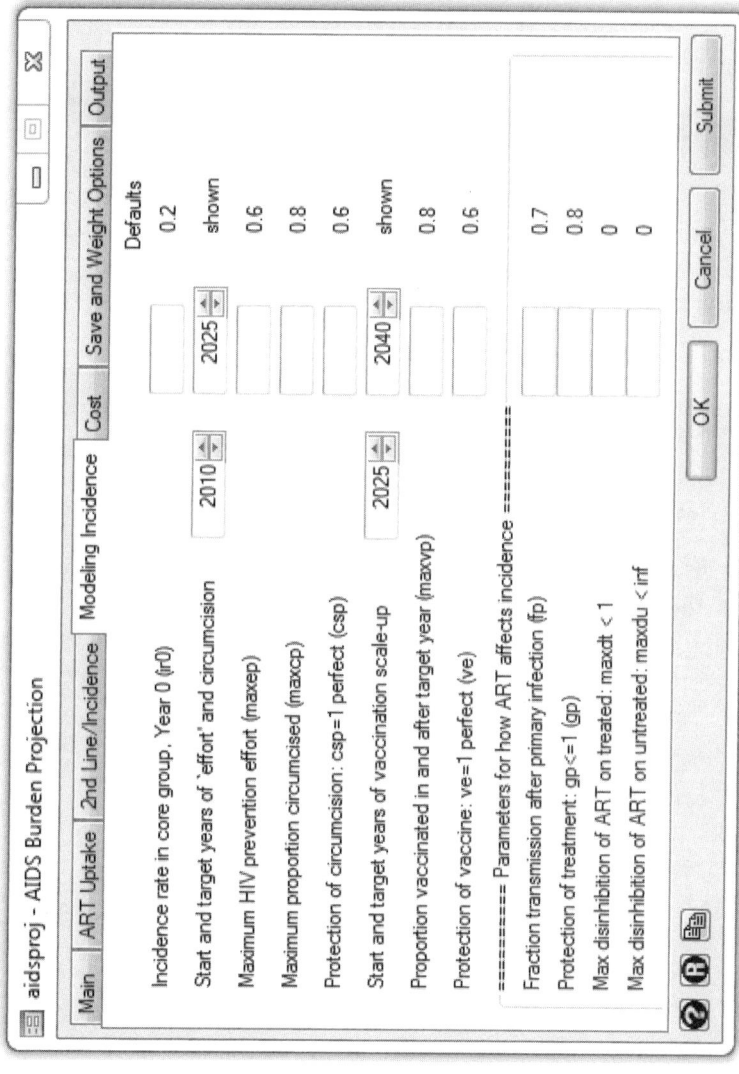

Source: Author's construction, available at www.cgdev.org/aidscost.

Notes

Notes to Chapter One

1. A note on terminology: HIV is a virus, or causal agent. AIDS is the collection of symptoms (or "syndrome") that occurs when the immune system begins to fail, typically about 10 years after infection. Although infectious, the patient is not sick until that point. The disease is best referred to as "HIV/AIDS" but sometimes just as "HIV" or "AIDS." The epidemic is formally called the "HIV/AIDS epidemic" but is sometimes informally referred to as either the "HIV epidemic" or the "AIDS epidemic." The phrase "people living with HIV/AIDS" is meant to include people who are infected with HIV but do not yet have any symptoms as well as those with symptoms and those whose symptoms are suppressed by treatment.

2. World Health Organization, "Fast facts on HIV/AIDS," www.who.int/hiv/data/fast_facts/en/index.html.

3. The WHO and UNAIDS do not report the number of persons initiating treatment in any year but only the number on treatment in each year. According to the WHO's September 2010 progress report, "[A]t the end of 2009, 5,254,000 people were receiving antiretroviral therapy in low- and middle-income countries, an increase of over 1.2 million people from December 2008" (WHO, UNAIDS, and UNICEF 2010, p. 51). Assuming that about 100,000 of those previously on treatment had died, and taking the November 2010 estimate from UNAIDS that there were 2.6 million new HIV infections in 2009 in low- and middle-income countries, the ratio of new treatment starts to new infections would be about one to two. This is only slightly better than the two-to-five ratio that the WHO and UNAIDS reported one year before.

4. The second chapter in this book discusses promising HIV-prevention opportunities.

5. Epidemiologists refer to the number of new infections as the incidence of HIV and the total number of infected people as the prevalence of HIV. The terms "prevalence" and "incidence" as epidemiologists use them correspond to what economists would call, respectively, the stock of current infections and the flow of new infections. The "prevalence rate" is defined as the proportion of a defined population, such as all adults aged 15 to 50, who are infected at a point in time, while the "incidence rate" is defined as the proportion of susceptible people who become infected during a year. Economists use the term "incidence" in an entirely different way to describe the distribution of a benefit or a cost across social groups. In this book, I adopt the epidemiologists' usage of the term "incidence."

6. See also Keith Montgomery, "The demographic transition," www.marathon. uwc.edu/geography/Demotrans/demtran.htm.

7. According to David Ho, who was first to recognize the extraordinary dynamics of HIV in the human body, the total virus production per day is somewhere between 1,010 and 1,012 virus particles. In a 2006 lecture, he said, "Half of [the virus particles] in circulation [in the bloodstream of an infected person] is removed in a half-hour, to be replaced by an equal amount of virus" (mitworld.mit.edu/video/360).

8. For example, evidence shows that among the HIV-negative spouses of ART patients, HIV infection rates are much smaller than among the HIV-negative spouses of HIV-infected people not on ART (Attia and others 2009; Granich and others 2009).

9. One possible explanation for increased risky behavior by people who have tested negative presumes that many of them know that they previously have had risky sexual contacts. Because public health messages rarely reveal that the probability of HIV transmission on a single sexual contact is less than one in twenty, those receiving negative test results experience cognitive dissonance between their belief that transmission is highly probable and their infection status. While one might resolve this dissonance by doubting the accuracy of a single negative test, after several negative tests, a person might logically conclude instead that he or she is, for some unknown reason, immune to HIV infection. Believing oneself to be immune then can logically justify riskier sexual activity. Another possible explanation for increased risky behavior after a negative test result is that the person who can claim such a result has more success in attracting partners.

10. According to data released in November 2010, new infections exceed deaths in 87 of 111, or 78 percent, of the low- and middle-income countries for which estimates are available (UNAIDS 2010).

11. The computer model used for these projections is open source and freely available for download so that readers can construct their own scenarios within the current structure of the program—or modify the program as desired. See Owen McCarthy and Mead Over, "Projecting the future budgetary cost of AIDS treatment (manual, software package, and dataset)," www.cgdev.org/content/ publications/detail/1422227/.

12. The "uptake rate" is distinct from the "coverage rate," defined as the total number of people receiving ART as a percentage of the total needing it. Both rates are measured with respect to a given definition of "need." In the following computations, a patient is assumed to need treatment when his or her CD4 count falls below 200 cells per microliter of blood.

13. These projections use the AIDSCost package described in annex c.

14. The 15 percent yearly uptake rate assigned to Nigeria is higher than its historical rate of 10 percent but required in order to hold mortality down.

15. Because a rate of incidence decline has never been observed in any of the three countries, this scenario seems reasonable.

16. One might argue that the planning horizon should be shorter because of technological uncertainty and myopic political decisionmaking—or that it should be even longer to capture more of the prevention benefits. My choice of a forty-year horizon is an admittedly arbitrary compromise between these views. Similarly, choosing too high a rate at which to discount future costs and benefits biases the analysis against prevention.

17. The model assumes subsidized cases in each country would converge to the target uptake rate over three years. The implication of this assumption is that with a zero uptake rate, an additional 1 million new patients would be added in 2011–2013 and no patients thereafter. This assumption is consistent with PEPFAR's stated objective of reaching 4 million patients by the year 2014. The model assumes treatment would have no effect on the rate of new infections. While recent research has highlighted the possibility that much more rapid and expensive treatment expansions than those considered here would slow transmission, the third chapter in this book discusses reasons the effect could go either way.

18. The total present value of the commitment is the amount of an endowment that, if established today, would just cover the costs of this commitment and be exhausted at the end of the forty-year period, assuming an interest rate of 3 percent over the period.

19. According to the Kaiser Family Foundation, total AIDS spending by all G8 donors in 2009 was $7.6 billion. I assume approximately half of this spending was on ART.

20. From 2007 to 2009, the typical sub-Saharan country's uptake rate was about 30 percent per year.

21. See note 18.

22. See note 18.

23. The third chapter in this book analyzes the benefits of increasing the threshold CD4 count at which patients are recruited to more closely approximate the new WHO recommendation that patients begin treatment when their CD4 count reaches 350 (WHO 2009). Since starting treatment earlier by raising this threshold expands the number needing treatment, the forty-year cost of any uptake rate would be larger than those displayed in figures 1-9 and 1-10.

24. Such a program is analogous with cap-and-trade proposals for limiting carbon dioxide emissions. Treatment programs that wish to recruit new patients could be asked to purchase a certain number of prevented HIV infections for every new treatment slot to be subsidized by the government or donors.

25. See Mead Over and David Wendt, "PEPFAR reauthorization IV: Target formula may unintentionally prevent improvements in PEPFAR implementation," Global Health Policy blog, August 4, 2008 (blogs.cgdev.org/globalhealth/2008/08/pepfar-reauthorization-iv-targ.php). The United States government belatedly met its legal obligation when it posted a summary of its cost studies on its website in July 2010 (see www.pepfar.gov/documents/organization/144993.pdf).

26. See www.pepfar.gov/documents/organization/133035.pdf for *The U.S. President's Emergency Plan for AIDS Relief: Five-Year Strategy*, published in 2009 by the Office of the United States Global AIDS Coordinator in collaboration with the Departments of State, Defense, Commerce, Labor, Health and Human Services, the U.S. Agency for International Development, and the Peace Corps.

27. Appendix A contains more detailed consideration of this option.

Notes to Chapter Two

1. The World Bank originally developed the DALY in order to measure each country's burden of disease (World Bank 1993). A country's "burden of disease" is defined as the number of DALYs per person that its population loses from all causes compared to the healthiest population in the world. In cost-effectiveness analysis, a reduction in DALYs lost constitutes an improvement in the population's health and thus is a measure of effectiveness that can be used to compare interventions across diseases.

2. Since each of the four randomized controlled trials of vaccines tested a biologically distinct vaccine, in a sense each trial is *sui generis*. The failure of three does not cast as much doubt on the validity of the one success as does the failure of eight trials in the case for the other success, STI treatment (Padian and others 2010). Despite the failed trials, many still believe that the treatment of curable STIs slows the rate of HIV infection, at least in an early stage of the epidemic, because HIV-infected people become more infectious when they also harbor a curable STI and because HIV-negative people with an STI have more CD4 cells in their genital tracts that are potential targets for invading HIV (Over and Piot 1996; Over and Aral 2006).

3. A late-breaking presentation at the Vienna AIDS conference in July 2010 showed that randomized controlled trials of a vaginal gel containing the antiretroviral medication tenofovir found statistically significant evidence that it effectively prevents HIV infection (Karim and others 2010). Administration via a vaginal gel is one of several ways that antiretroviral medications could be used to prevent HIV infection. This class of prevention strategies is referred to as pre-exposure prophylaxis and is the subject of considerable speculation. Note, however, that use of anti-

retroviral agents for this class of prevention will compete with, and thus exacerbate the scarcity of, these medications in their primary use of treating AIDS patients.

4. Conditional payments to governments are also a promising way to improve HIV prevention. Such policies are explored at the end of this chapter.

5. Preliminary results from a follow-up study that Thornton conducted in Malawi suggest that offering a payment to HIV-negative people for remaining negative is not a sufficient—or a sufficiently plausible—prevention incentive.

6. The results of this randomized trial are encouraging in another respect: they refute the assertion that poor African women have little or no physical control over their own sexual risk. Another randomized study shows that when young, poor African women are informed that older men are more likely to be HIV infected, they reduce the frequency with which they have sex with older men (Dupas 2010).

7. See World Bank, "Malawi and Tanzania research shows promise in preventing HIV and sexually-transmitted infections," press release, July 18, 2010 (go. worldbank.org/YVMPZBKC00).

8. Sensitivity assumes longer coverage of those targeted and thus improved total benefit. Specificity improves cost-effectiveness because it enables a closer match between the message and incentives offered with the circumstances of the targeted individuals.

9. The challenge for the modelers, on the other hand, is to incorporate the concept of channels in their models to test the robustness of their cost-effectiveness results in this more realistic framework. When modelers are able to calibrate the parameters of channel effectiveness from the data prevention implementers collect, quantitative prediction of future HIV-infection rates will be able to support an AIDS transition strategy.

10. A four-year follow-up of the Uganda case shows a 75 percent reduction in HIV incidence in men who were circumcised compared to those who elected not to undergo circumcision. If this strengthened effect is confirmed by other studies, it will be interesting to know if apparently improved results over a longer follow-up period are because of attrition or selection bias or if circumcision's benefits for any individual improve over time. See Ron Gray's comment to Mead Over, "Adult male circumcision as an HIV prevention tool: Should the scale up of an efficacious intervention be evaluated?" Global Health Policy blog, January 26, 2010 (blogs.cgdev.org/global health/2010/01/adult-male-circumcision-as-an-hiv-prevention-tool-should-the-scale up-of-an-efficacious-intervention-be-evaluated.php).

11. See Potts and others (2008) for a brief review of recent male circumcision studies.

12. There are three possible outcomes of couples testing: partners who are concordant negative (both are HIV negative), concordant positive, and discordant. In concordant negative partnerships, which are most common at younger ages (Beegle and de Walque 2009), full information achieved through couples testing unequivocally strengthens the incentive to remain faithful to the partnership because each partner faces greater risk with an outside partner of unknown HIV status.

13. There is anecdotal evidence that such counterfeit certificates are already in circulation. See, for example, Peter Emeka Nwafor, "HIV AIDS and Nigerian settlers in South Africa: matters arising" (nigeriaworld.com/articles/2010/jun/282.htm).

14. The statistic for Rwanda comes from Allen's unpublished data from more than 5,000 couple-years of follow-up between 2003 and 2009.

15. Participants at a WHO-sponsored workshop on November 9, 2009, made these points and others suggesting the fragility of the WHO group's results. See www.who.int/hiv/topics/artforprevention/modelling_meeting/en/index.html.

16. For more discussion of the potential contributions of adherence support organizations and the cost of running them, see the third chapter in this book and Revenga and others 2006.

17. This account is from Kevin Palmer of the World Health Organization, whom the author interviewed in 2010.

18. After Argentina entered into World Bank–funded, performance-based contracts with its provinces in 2004 regarding ten indicators of maternal and child health, a study found that the provinces actively sought "technical assistance to improve information systems, expand enrollment, and contract and pay providers" (Eichler and Glassman 2008, p. 13).

19. This section of this chapter draws heavily on work by Hallett and Over (2010).

20. For example, according to UNAIDS, only about three-quarters of patients who enroll in ART are retained for two years in the same program (WHO, UNAIDS, and UNICEF 2009). The larger the number of these disappearing patients who successfully re-enroll elsewhere, rather than succumb to the disease, the greater will be the prevalence of HIV in the population in the counterfactual—and vice versa. A higher counterfactual prevalence, when compared to any observed prevalence, will lead to a larger estimate of prevalence reduction and thus a greater COD payout. Thus, modelers will be under pressure from the recipient government to assume that most disappearing patients successfully find new treatment options in order to bias the measurement toward a higher payment.

21. Evidence suggests that these tests can misclassify two types of people as recently infected: the unusually sick whose immune systems are greatly impaired and the unexpectedly healthy whose immune systems have effectively suppressed the infection for years.

22. Tests similar to those used to track a patient's immune system during ART can determine whether an individual who scores positively on a TRI might be misclassified owing to either a disabled immune system or an exceptionally effective one.

23. Some modeling still might be necessary to best arrive at an incidence measurement after combining the information from several tests.

24. In other words, two samples of 8,000 yield a statistical power of 80 percent for the test that prevalence has declined in this hypothetical model. A test of this hypothesis with this power would ordinarily require only that the two samples be of 730 persons each. The requirements of the prevalence modeling approach, however, push the sample size requirement up to 8,000.

25. The same power could be attained with two samples of only 12,500 each if the interval between surveys increases to six years.

26. For example, suppose that a particular sample is unlucky in the direction of overestimating incidence leading to a reduction in the payout. The next time a survey is conducted, it is unlikely to be unlucky in the same direction. If it is more accurate, the difference in incidence between the preceding survey and this new one will be biased upward. Thus the payout foregone on the first iteration of the COD program would be made up by an overpayment on the second iteration. As the iterations of the program accumulate, the law of large numbers guarantees that the total accumulated payment will converge to the amount that properly rewards the actual accomplishment.

27. Some observers might see such a market-like mechanism as a threat to the aid allocation they would have preferred. But recognizing donors' right to select which of multiple gifts they prefer to give is a plausible alternative to bureaucratically planned foreign aid programs—and might elicit a greater total amount of donor financing.

28. Although their application is to primary-school completion, an area where human rights abuses seem less likely, Birdsall and Savedoff (2010) discuss the possibility of incorporating a "social audit" into their model COD contract as protection against unintended consequences.

29. Analysis of the interviewer codes recorded in the data from a household seroprevalence survey in Namibia revealed the strong probability that a single interviewer had provided samples of his own blood in lieu of visiting and taking blood from members of the households that were the object of research (Janssens and others 2009; Janssens, van der Gaag, and Rinke de-Wit 2009).

30. Economists use a discount rate to reduce the value of future costs and benefits compared to current ones. For example, at a discount rate of 100 percent, only the current year's treatment cost would matter to a decisionmaker because all future costs would be entirely discounted. In the belief that a responsible government should plan responsibly for the future, even weighing the well-being of the unborn in its current calculations, economists typically recommend a low discount rate to government decisionmakers. The World Bank (1993) adopted the rate of 3 percent for evaluating future health benefits and losses in its *1993 World Development Report*, and this rate has since become conventional in the analysis of future health benefits and their associated costs. An even lower discount rate would yield larger estimates of the present value of a stream of future treatment costs.

Notes to Chapter Three

1. Quote appears in paragraph 18D in the section of the G-8 Communiqué on Africa titled "Investing in People" (www.g8.utoronto.ca/summit/2005gleneagles/communique.pdf).

2. Office of U.S. Global AIDS Coordinator, "Latest Results" (www.pepfar.gov/results/index.htm, accessed April 4, 2011).

3. The definition of "needing treatment" continues to change. An important measure of the progression of HIV is the number of CD4 counts per milliliter of a patient's blood, a count that declines from close to a thousand for an uninfected person to zero as HIV destroys a person's immune system. After years of consensus that the threshold for AIDS treatment should be 200 cells per microliter (WHO 2006)—about eight years after HIV infection—evidence is accumulating that starting treatment a year or more earlier, when the CD4 count is 350, would improve the effectiveness of treatment (When to Start Consortium and Sterne 2009). The WHO revised its guidelines on December 1, 2009, to recommend beginning treatment at a CD4 count of 350. These revised coverage percentages appear in a 2010 progress report by WHO, UNAIDS, and UNICEF (2010).

4. The 2003 PEPFAR authorization required that 55 percent of expenditures be on AIDS treatment; the 2008 re-authorization reduced that minimum to 50 percent.

5. Farah Stockman, "US Seeks to Rein in AIDS Program," *Boston Globe*, April 11, 2010 (www.boston.com/news/nation/washington/articles/2010/04/11/us_seeks_to_rein_in_aids_program/).

6. "Replenishing the fund: finding the money to fight AIDS," September 26, 2007, www.economist.com/node/9860562.

7. These fifteen countries were Botswana, Côte d'Ivoire, Ethiopia, Guyana, Haiti, Kenya, Mozambique, Namibia, Nigeria, Rwanda, South Africa, Tanzania, Uganda, Vietnam, and Zambia. In January 2011, PEPFAR reported the number of AIDS patients whose treatment it directly supports from the above countries and also Cambodia, China, Democratic Republic of the Congo, India, Lesotho, Russia, Swaziland, Thailand, and Zimbabwe, for a total of twenty-four countries receiving direct support.

8. For example, AIDS patients or their governments could begin to resent their dependency. Elsewhere, I have suggested that the situation where citizens in a poor country are dependent on the benevolence of foreign donors for their day-to-day existence might be characterized as "post-modern colonialism" (Over 2008).

9. On September 26, 2007, UNAIDS (The Joint United Nations Program on HIV/AIDS) requested $50 billion a year in AIDS funding, up from the current level of about $10 billion a year from all sources. Of this current amount, $7.6 is from the G-8 donors and the rest is from private philanthropy (UNAIDS 2007).

10. A 2002 World Bank study in support of the Millennium Development Goals estimated that the cost of achieving all eight of the goals by the year 2015 would be between $40 and $60 billion per year (Devarajan, Miller, and Swanson 2002).

11. According to Reuters's Mathew Bunce, "French President Jacques Chirac addressed Africa's top AIDS conference . . . and called on the world's richest nations to create an AIDS therapy support fund to help Africa. According to Chirac, Africa struggles to care for two-thirds of the world's persons with AIDS without the benefit of expensive AIDS therapies. Chirac invited other countries, especially European nations, to create a fund that would help increase the number of AIDS studies and experiments. AIDS workers welcomed Chirac's speech and said they hoped France

would promote the idea to the Group of Eight summit of the world's richest nations." See Matthew Bunce, "France's Chirac Calls for AIDS Therapy Fund," Reuters, December 7, 1997 (www.aegis.com/news/ads/1997/AD972244.html).

12. What I call the "uptake rate" has also been called the "enrollment ratio" (Johnson and Boulle 2011).

13. Depending on their drug regimes and their individual sensitivity to those drugs, some patients experience alterations in weight or appearance due to the atrophy or displacement of fat deposits in their face, back, or abdomen. One Thai patient in a focus group interview said, "I am confused about ART. I do not understand why my weight went up and I am disturbed by the fact that the fat growth is misplaced. If I could go back, I would not join ART until my health was at its worst" (Revenga and others 2006, 6).

14. The hypothesis that the growth rate of HIV/AIDS assistance in 1999 does not change can be rejected at a p-value of 10-8.

15. For non-HIV/AIDS health assistance, the point estimate of the growth rate from 1999 to 2007 is 7.4 percent, slightly higher than the 5.8 percent rate estimated prior to 1999. But the p-value on the test of a change in the trend in 1999 is 0.06, greater than the conventional threshold for statistical significance of 0.05.

16. "CGD hosts Secretary Clinton address: 'Development assistance in the 21st century,'" Center for Global Development press release, January 6, 2010, www.cgdev.org/content/general/detail/1423520.

17. Because monotherapy with AZT and imperfect adherence slow but do not completely suppress viral reproduction, a descendent of the original virus eventually appears that by chance is resistant to that drug and then is able to reproduce, crowding out the other genetic variants and leading to treatment failure in that patient. Drug resistance is an example of Darwinian selection operating at "warp speed" within the body of a single patient.

18. The seventeen Latin-American countries in the survey use more heterogeneous drug combinations (UNAIDS 2010, page 66).

19. When a country is unaware of prices other countries pay for a drug, its negotiators are in a weak position relative to the representatives of pharmaceutical manufacturers or suppliers and therefore may agree to pay a higher price than the seller would be willing to accept. The advent of the WHO's Global Price Reporting Mechanism, supported by the Price Reporting Mechanism at the Global Fund for AIDS, Tuberculosis and Malaria, has improved the availability of price information and therefore may have contributed directly to the price reductions shown in Figure 3-7.

20. The International AIDS Society (2009) defines "universal access" as treatment for 80 percent of those in need. UNAIDS allows each country to define its own targets. The most modest definition is that of Mozambique, which for 2010 defined "universal" to mean 45 percent.

21. Henry J. Kaiser Family Foundation, "International AIDS Assistance: Trends in G8/EC & Other Donor Assistance, 2002–2009" (facts.kff.org/chart.aspx?ch=946).

22. With this ambitious treatment expansion, the unmet need for ART will decline rapidly, as will the "funding gap"—that is, the cost of providing treatment for the other 20 percent of those who need care.

23. Organization for Economic Cooperation and Development, "Total DAC countries" (www.oecd.org/dataoecd/17/39/44285701.gif).

24. Other assumptions for Figures 3-8 and 3-9 include that median CD4 count at recruitment is unchanged at 130, second-line therapy coverage reaches 95 percent by the year 2020, and the elasticity of average fixed cost with respect to scale is –0.146. In a newer version of the AIDSCost model constructed jointly with Geoffrey Garnett of Imperial College, we assume that the incidence rate would remain a constant fraction of the susceptible adult population but could be reduced by ART or male circumcision. In this model even full coverage of ART and circumcision are insufficient to reduce incidence lower than annual mortality and the annual cost of AIDS treatment rises to $150 billion by the year 2050.

25. Years on second-line treatment cost more than those on first-line treatment. Since late recruitment entails a greater likelihood of the failure of first-line treatment, it would incur greater costs per patient-year, but this cost-increasing effect is offset by the cost-decreasing effect of higher mortality with earlier recruitment. Furthermore, the short period until 2014 does not allow enough time for many patients to move to second-line treatment. So within this framework, patient-years of treatment cost roughly the same at all uptake and initiation CD4 counts.

26. A previous version of this analysis appeared in Mead Over, "How Will PEPFAR Reach 4 Million AIDS Patients on Treatment by 2014: Expanded Access or Earlier Recruitment? Millions of Years of Life Hang in the Balance," Global Health Policy blog, December 8, 2009 (blogs.cgdev.org/globalhealth/2009/12/how-will-pepfar-reach-4-million-aids-patients-on-treatment-by-2014-expanded-access-or-earlier-recruitment-millions-of-years-of-life-hang-in-the-balance.php).

27. The calculations in this book assume that second-line coverage increases gradually from the regional average given by the WHO to 95 percent coverage by the year 2020.

28. This section draws on Over 2009a.

29. The situation is actually a bit more complex. Since people have insurance and precautionary saving, some out-of-pocket payments are pre-financed and therefore should not be seen as causing immiseration. This pre-financed proportion should instead be subtracted from both gross and net consumption. Such a shift could move an individual who appears to be impoverished by health care expenditures to a position from which health expenditure no longer pushes him or her below the poverty line. For in-depth discussion, see Wagstaff, Van Doorslaer, and Paci 1989; Van Doorslaer, Wagstaff, and Rutten 1993; Wagstaff 2002; and Van Doorslaer, O'Donell, and others 2007.

30. An early challenge to the assumption that HIV prevalence would be higher among poor or uneducated people is presented in Ainsworth and Over 1997. The incorporation of blood tests into general-purpose national surveys has shown that

the highest HIV prevalence levels are often at the middle or even the highest levels of socioeconomic status in African countries (Barnighausen and others 2007; Montana, Mishra, and Hong 2008).

31. Over and others (2004) model the possible benefits from public-sector crowding out of lower-quality private-sector ART in India.

32. For a fuller discussion of performance-based incentives, see chapter 2.

33. This idea was first suggested in a study of the economics of AIDS treatment in Thailand. The authors gave an example of an affinity group of AIDS patients that not only supported its members to ensure they understood the providers' instructions but also helped their members carry out those instructions (Revenga and others 2006). This group also spent several evenings a month conducting HIV-prevention outreach in the bars and brothels of Phuket.

34. For a more on COD, particularly for prevention, see chapter 2.

35. See Institute of Medicine 2007 and Over 2008, 2009b for suggestions that the U.S. PEPFAR program has focused excessively on increasing the number of patients on treatment regardless of their success at remaining on treatment.

Notes to Appendixes

1. On the costs of HIV-prevention activities, see Guinness and others 2005; Guinness, Kumaranayake, and Hanson 2007; Kumaranayake and Watts 2000; Marseille and others 2007. For ART, researchers have undertaken individual cost studies, but unfortunately no one has yet published data on a large enough range of study sites to permit estimation of economies of scale (Cleary, McIntyre, and Boulle 2006; Over and others 2006; Over and others 2007; Leisegang and others 2009; Nachega and others 2010). Although the 2008 President's Emergency Plan for AIDS Relief (PEPFAR) authorization bill mandates that by September 30, 2009, the U.S. administration provide to Congress studies that estimate the unit cost of ART, at the time of this writing the administration has not yet fully complied with this mandate. See discussions of the implication of the mandate by Menzies and others (Forthcoming); Walker, Over, and Bertozzi (Forthcoming); and in Mead Over, "PEPFAR Reauthorization IV: Target Formula May Unintentionally Prevent Improvements in PEPFAR Implementation," Global Health Policy blog, August 4, 2008 (http://blogs.cgdev.org/globalhealth/2008/08/pepfar-reauthorization-iv-targ.php).

2. UNGASS is the acronym for the United Nations General Assembly Special Session on HIV/AIDS, which occurred June 25–27, 2001, in New York City. This session established a set of indicators that member countries would report to UNAIDS each year.

3. This is the source of the figures in row h of table 3-1 in the text.

4. For a fuller discussion of future drug prices, see page 106.

5. In an attempt to achieve treatment coverage close to 100 percent, average costs would likely rise due to the requirement that treatment facilities be located in small communities, where the small numbers of patients would prevent economies

of scale. Because donors are unlikely to finance such high treatment coverage rates, partly for exactly this reason, the models in this book do not incorporate these eventual scale diseconomies.

6. The fitted trend line in figure B-1 is linear in logarithms. The slope of a function that is linear in logarithms is referred to by economists as an "elasticity" and has the virtue of being unit free. It gives the percentage change of the dependent variable associated with a 1 percent change of the independent variable. In this case, the estimated elasticity is -0.39.

7. My method for estimating mortality among the patients lost to follow-up is to choose the value of that mortality that maximizes the goodness of fit of the log-linear regression of mortality on CD4 at initiation. The best-fitting value is 60 percent mortality among those lost to follow-up, which yields the upper of the two mortality curves in figure B-2 (Fox, McCarthy, and Over 2011). By assigning this mortality rate to those who start ART, I implicitly assume that the attrition from treatment programs will remain constant across the various scenarios under consideration.

8. Dividing the no-ART hazard rates from the curve fitted to the ART-linc study data by the When to Start Consortium hazard ratios generates the triangle points in figure B-2. The graph shows that these triangles converge to the adjusted no-ART mortality at low CD4 counts, thus tying together all three data sources (eART-linc 2008; When to Start Consortium and 2009; Fox, McCarthy, and Over 2011) and supporting the proposition that the high-income country hazard ratios can be applied plausibly to the low-income country no-ART hazard rates.

9. See White 2007 for discussion of appropriate parameter values for the model and the Spectrum projection model for an alternative modeling platform (www.futuresinstitute.org/). On cost assumptions, see Bollinger, Stover, and UNAIDS 2007.

10. A reference manual and user's guide for this software is available at www.CGDev.org. Users with a copy of Stata can find and install the software by typing the phrase "findit AIDSCost" (omitting quotation marks but respecting the capitalization) in the Stata command window.

References

Ainsworth, M., and A. M. Over. 1997. *Confronting AIDS: Public Priorities in a Global Epidemic.* Oxford University Press.

Akerloff, George A. 1970. "The Market for 'Lemons': Quality Uncertainty and the Market Mechanism." *Quarterly Journal of Economics* 84 (3) (August): 488–500.

Alary, M., and others. 2010. "Ecological analysis of the association between high-risk population parameters and HIV prevalence among pregnant women enrolled in sentinel surveillance in four Southern India states." *Sexually Transmitted Infections* 86 (Supplement 1): i10–i16.

Allen, S. 2010. "Cost of averting HIV infections in Africa: voluntary HIV counseling and testing for couples (CVCT) vs. ARV-as-prevention ('test-and-treat' (TNT))." Presentation at the Center for Global Development. Washington, DC, June 8, 2010. www.cgdev.org/doc/events/06.08.10/FinalAllenCGDJune2010rev2.pdf

Allen, S., A. Serufilira, J. Bogaerts, and others. 1992. "Confidential HIV testing and condom promotion in Africa. Impact on HIV and gonorrhea rates." *JAMA: The Journal of the American Medical Association* 268 (23): 3338–3343.

Allen, S., A. Serufilira, V. Gruber, and others. 1993. "Pregnancy and contraception use among urban Rwandan women after HIV testing and counseling." *American Journal of Public Health* 83 (5): 705–707.

Allen, S., J. Tice, and others. 1992. "Effect of serotesting with counselling on condom use and seroconversion among HIV discordant couples in Africa." *British Medical Journal* 304 (6842): 1605–1609.

Atkinson, J. A., and others. 2010. "Community participation for malaria elimination in Tafea Province, Vanuatu: Part I. Maintaining motivation for prevention practices in the context of disappearing disease." *Malaria Journal* 9.

Attia, S., and others. 2009. "Sexual transmission of HIV according to viral load and antiretroviral therapy: systematic review and meta-analysis." *AIDS* 23 (11): 1397–1404.

Auvert, B., and others. 2005. "Randomized, controlled intervention trial of male circumcision for reduction of HIV infection risk: the ANRS 1265 Trial." *PLoSMedicine* 2 (11): e298.

Bailey, R. C., and others. 2007. "Male circumcision for HIV prevention in young men in Kisumu, Kenya: a randomised controlled trial." *Lancet* 369 (9562): 643–656.

Baird, S., and others. 2010. "The short-term impacts of a schooling conditional cash transfer program on the sexual behavior of young women." *Health Economics* 19 (Supplement 1): 55–68.

Bangsberg, D. R., and others. 2003. "High levels of adherence do not prevent accumulation of HIV drug resistance mutations." *AIDS* 17 (13): 1925–1932.

Barder, O., and N. Birdsall. 2006. "Payments for Progress: A Hands-Off Approach to Foreign Aid." Working Paper 102. Center for Global - Development.

Barnighausen, T., and others. 2007. "The socioeconomic determinants of HIV incidence: evidence from a longitudinal, population-based study in rural South Africa." *AIDS* 21 (Supplement 7): S29–S38.

Bautista-Arredondo, S., and others. 2008. "Optimizing resource allocation for HIV/AIDS prevention programmes: an analytical framework." *AIDS* 22 (Supplement 1): S67–S74.

Beegle, K., and D. de Walque. 2009. "Demographic and socioeconomic patterns of HIV/AIDS prevalence in Africa." Policy Research Working Paper 5076. World Bank.

Bertozzi, S. M., N. Padian, and T. E. Martz. 2010. "Evaluation of HIV prevention programmes: the case of Avahan." *Sexually Transmitted Infections* 86 (Supplement 1): i4–i5.

Bill & Melinda Gates Foundation. 2010. *Treat and Prevent: Avahan's Experience in Scaling Up STI Services to Groups at High Risk of HIV Infection in India.*

Birdsall, N., and W. Savedoff. 2010. *Cash on Delivery: A New Approach to Foreign Aid, with an Application to Primary Schooling.* Brookings.

Bloom, D. E., and J. G. Williamson. 1998. "Demographic Transitions and Economic Miracles in Emerging Asia." *World Bank Economic Review* 12 (3): 419–455.

Bollinger, L., J. Stover, and UNAIDS. 2007. "Methodology for care and treatment interventions." In *Financial Resources Required to Achieve Universal Access to HIV, Prevention, Treatment, Care and Support.* The Joint United Nations Program on HIV/AIDS (UNAIDS), AnnexIII. data.unaids.org/pub/Report/2007/20070925_annex_iii_treatment_care_methodology_en.pdf.

Bongaarts, J., and others. 1989. "The relationship between male circumcision and HIV infection in African populations." *AIDS* 3 (6): 373–377.

Brinkhof, M. W., M. Pujades-Rodriguez, and M. Egger. 2009. "Mortality of patients lost to follow-up in antiretroviral treatment programmes in resource-limited settings: systematic review and meta-analysis." *PLoS ONE* 4 (6): e5790.

Case, A. 2009. "The impact of HIV on marriage patterns in sub-Saharan Africa." Presentation to Amsterdam Institute for International Development annual workshops, "Economic Consequences of AIDS." Amsterdam, December 18–19.

Chaisson, R., and others. 1996. "Effects of an incentive and education program on return rates for PPD test reading in patients with HIV infection." *Journal of Acquired Immune Deficiency Syndrome and Human Retrovirology* 11 (5): 455–459.

Cleary, S. M., D. McIntyre, and A. M. Boulle. 2006. "The cost-effectiveness of antiretroviral treatment in Khayelitsha, South Africa—a primary data analysis." *Cost Effectivness and Resource Allocation* 4: 20.

Clemens, M. 2007. "Do visas kill? Health effects of African health professional emigration." Working Paper 114. Center for Global Development.

Coale, A. J. 1973. "The Demographic Transition." In *Congrès International de la Population, Vol. I.* International Union for the Scientific Study of Population, 53–71.

Dandona, L., P. Sisodia, S. G. Prem Kumar, and others. 2005. "HIV prevention programmes for female sex workers in Andhra Pradesh, India: outputs, cost and efficiency." *BMC Public Health* 5: 98.

Dandona, L., P. Sisodia, T. L. N. Prasad, and others. 2005. "Cost and efficiency of public sector sexually transmitted infection clinics in Andhra Pradesh, India." *BMC Health Services Research* 5: 69.

Dandona, L., Y. K. Ramesh, and others. 2005. "Cost and efficiency of HIV voluntary counselling and testing centres in Andhra Pradesh, India." *National Medical Journal of India* 18: 26–31.

Deaton, Angus S. 2009. "Instruments of development: randomization in the tropics, and the search for the elusive keys to economic development." Working Paper 14690. National Bureau of Economic Research.

Devarajan, S., M. J. Miller, and E. V. Swanson. 2002. "Goals for development: history, prospects, and costs." Working Paper 2819. World Bank, Human Development Network, Office of the Vice President, and Development Data Group.

de Walque, D., H. Kazianga, and M. A. Over. 2010. "Antiretroviral therapy awareness and risky sexual behaviors: evidence from Mozambique." Working Paper 5486. World Bank.

Dodd, P. J., G. P. Garnett, and T. B. Hallett. 2010. "Examining the promise of HIV elimination by 'test and treat' in hyperendemic settings." *AIDS* 24 (5): 729–735.

Dunkle, K. L., and others. 2008. "New heterosexually transmitted HIV infections in married or cohabiting couples in urban Zambia and Rwanda: an analysis of survey and clinical data." *Lancet* 371 (9631): 2183–2191.

Dupas, P. 2010. "Do teenagers respond to HIV risk information? Evidence from an HIV field experiment in Kenya." Working paper 14707. National Bureau of Economic Research. www.nber.org/papers/w14707.

eART-linc. 2008. "Duration from seroconversion to eligibility for antiretroviral therapy and from ART eligibility to death in adult HIV-infected patients from low and middle-income countries; collaborative analysis of prospective studies." *Sexually Transmitted Infections* 84 (Supplement 1): 31–36.

Easterly, W. 2006. *The White Man's Burden: Why the West's Efforts to Aid Africa Have Done So Much Ill and So Little Good.* Penguin Group.

Eichler, R., and A. Glassman. 2008. "Health systems strengthening via performance-based aid: Creating incentives to perform and to measure results." Global Health Financing Initiative Working Paper 3. Brookings.

Eichler, R., R. Levine, and Performance-Based Incentives Working Group. 2009. *Performance Incentives for Global Health: Potential and Pitfalls.* Brookings Institution Press.

Epstein, H. 2007. *The Invisible Cure: Africa, the West, and the Fight Against AIDS.* Farrar, Straus and Giroux.

Evaluation Gap Working Group. 2006. *When Will We Ever Learn? Improving Lives through Impact Evaluation.* Center for Global Development.

Farquhar, C., and others. 2004. "Antenatal couple counseling increases uptake of interventions to prevent HIV-1 transmission." *Journal of Acquired Immune Deficiency Syndromes* 37 (5): 1620–1626.

Fideli, U. S., and others. 2001. "Virologic and immunologic determinants of heterosexual transmission of human immunodeficiency virus type 1 in Africa." *AIDS Research and Human Retroviruses* 17 (10): 901–910.

Filmer, D., and L. Pritchett. 1999. "The impact of public spending on health: does money matter?" *Social Science &Medicine* 49 (10): 1309–1323.

Fox, M. P., O. F. McCarthy, and M. A. Over. 2011. "A meta-analytic approach to estimating the relation between initiating CD4 count and mortality using a novel method of adjusting for loss to follow up." Unpublished paper. Center for Global Development and Boston University.

Fox, M. P., and S. Rosen. 2010. "Systematic review of patient retention in antiretroviral therapy programs up to three years on treatment in sub-Saharan Africa, 2007–2009." *Tropical Medicine and International Health* 1 (Supplement 1): 1–15.

Friedland, G. H., and A. Williams. 1999. "Attaining higher goals in HIV treatment: the central importance of adherence." *AIDS* 13 (Supplement 1): 61–72.

Galarraga, O., and others. 2009. "HIV prevention cost-effectiveness: a systematic review." *BMC Public Health* 9 (Supplement 1): S5.

Garnett, Geoffrey P., and others. 2010. "Patterns of self-reported behaviour change associated with receiving voluntary counselling and testing in a longitudinal study from Manicaland, Zimbabwe." *AIDS and Behavior* 14, no. 3: 708–15.

Gertler, P., and others. 2009. "Paying health care providers for performance: evidence from Rwanda." Presentation at the Economics Reference Group meeting, "Sustaining HIV Prevention and Treatment." Washington, DC, April 21–22. www.heard.org.za/research/economics-reference-group/fifth-meeting.

Ghys, P. D., and others. 2010. "Trends in HIV prevalence and sexual behaviour among young people aged 15–24 years in countries most affected by HIV." *Sexually Transmitted Infections* 86 (Supplement 2): ii72–ii83.

Golladay, F. L., and others. 1976. "Policy planning for the mid-level health worker: economic potentials and barriers to change." *Inquiry* 13 (1): 80–89.

Granich, R. M., and others. 2009. "Universal voluntary HIV testing with immediate antiretroviral therapy as a strategy for elimination of HIV transmission: a mathematical model." *Lancet* 373 (9657): 48–57.

Gray, R., and others. 2007. "Male circumcision for HIV prevention in men in Rakai, Uganda: a randomised trial." *Lancet* 369 (9562): 657–666.

Guinness, L., L. Kumaranayake, and K. Hanson. 2007. "A cost function for HIV prevention services: is there a 'u' - shape?" *Cost Effectivness and Resource Allocation* 5: 13.

Guinness, L., and others. 2005. "Does scale matter? The costs of HIV-prevention interventions for commercial sex workers in India." *Bulletin of the World Health Organization* 83 (10): 747–755.

Guwatudde. D., and others. 2009. "Relatively low HIV infection rates in rural Uganda, but with high potential for a rise: a cohort study in Kayunga District, Uganda." *PLoS ONE* 4, no. 1: e4145.

Hallett, T. B., and M. Over. 2010. "How to pay 'cash-on-delivery' for HIV infections averted: two measurement approaches and ten payout functions." Working Paper 210. Center for Global Development.

Hallett, T. B., and others. 2006. "Declines in HIV prevalence can be associated with changing sexual behaviour in Uganda, urban Kenya, Zimbabwe, and urban Haiti." *Sexually Transmitted Infections* 82 (Supplement 1): i1–i8.

Hallett, T. B., S. Gregson, and others. 2009. "Assessing evidence for behaviour change affecting the course of HIV epidemics: a new mathematical modelling approach and application to data from Zimbabwe." *Epidemics* 1 (2): 108–117.

Halperin, D. T., and H. Epstein. 2004. "Concurrent sexual partnerships help to explain Africa's high HIV prevalence: implications for prevention." *Lancet* 364 (9428): 4–6.

Hammer, S. M., and others. 2008. "Antiretroviral treatment of adult HIV infection: 2008 recommendations of the International AIDS Society-USA panel." *JAMA: The Journal of the American Medical Association* 300 (5): 555–570.

Hethecote, H. W., and J. A. Yorke. 1984. *Gonorrhea Transmission Control and Dynamics*. Springer-Levin.

Hira, S. K., and others. 1990. "Epidemiology of human immunodeficiency virus in families in Lusaka, Zambia."*Journal of Acquired Immune Deficiency Syndromes* 3 (1): 83–86.

Hogan, D. R., and others. 2005. "Cost effectiveness analysis of strategies to combat HIV/AIDS in developing countries." *British Medical Journal* 331: 1431.

Holmes, C. B., and others. 2010. "Use of generic antiretroviral agents and cost savings in PEPFAR treatment programs."*JAMA* 304 (3): 313–320.

Institute of Medicine. 2007. *PEPFAR Implementation: Progress and Promise*. National Academies Press.

International AIDS Society. 2009. "Reaffirming the G8 commitment to universal access: Gleneagles + five." Backgrounder. www.iasociety.org/Web/WebContent/File/IAS_GC%20Backgrounder_%2019%20Nov%2020 09.pdf.

Janssens, W., J. van der Gaag, and T. Rinke de-Wit. 2009. "Refusal bias in the estimation of HIV prevalence." Research series 08-03. University of Amsterdam, Amsterdam Institute for International Development.

Janssens, W., and others. 2009. "A cautious note on household survey HIV prevalence estimates in Africa."Research series 10-08. University of Amsterdam, Amsterdam Institute for International Development.

Johnson, L. F., and A. Boulle. 2011. "How should access to antiretroviral treatment be measured?"*Bulletin of the World Health Organization* 89: 157–160.

Kaneko, A. 2010. "A community-directed strategy for sustainable malaria elimination on islands: short-term MDA integrated with ITNs and robust surveillance." *Acta Trop* 114 (3): 177–183.

Kaneko, A., and others. 2000. "Malaria eradication on islands." *The Lancet* 356 (9241): 1560–1564.

Karim, Q. A., and others. 2010. "Effectiveness and safety of tenofovir gel, an antiretroviral microbicide, for the prevention of HIV infection in women." *Science* 329 (5996): 1168–1174.

Katz, M. H., and others. 2002. "Impact of highly active antiretroviral treatment on HIV seroincidence among men who have sex with men: San Francisco." *American Journal of Public Health* 92 (3): 388–394.

Katzenstein, D., M. Laga, and J. P. Moatti. 2003. "The evaluation of the HIV/AIDS drug access initiatives in Côted'Ivoire, Senegal and Uganda: how access to antiretroviral treatment can become feasible in Africa." *AIDS* 17 (Supplement 3): S1–S4.

Kempf, M. C., and others. 2008. "Enrollment and retention of HIV discordant couples in Lusaka, Zambia." *Journal of Acquired Immune Deficiency Syndromes* 47 (1): 116–125.

Kumaranayake, L., and C. Watts. 2000. "Economic costs of HIV/AIDS prevention activities in sub-Saharan Africa." *AIDS* 14 (Supplement 3): S239–S252.

Lagakos, S. W., and A. R. Gable. 2008. "Challenges to HIV prevention— seeking effective measures in the absence of a vaccine." *New England Journal of Medicine* 358 (15): 1543–1545.

Leisegang, R., and others. 2009. "Early and late direct costs in a Southern African antiretroviral treatment programme: a retrospective cohort analysis." *PLoS. Medicine* 6 (12): e1000189.

Lyman, P. N. and S. B. Wittels. 2010. "No good deed goes unpunished." *Foreign Affairs* 89 (4): 74–84.

Marseille, E., and others. 2004. "Assessing the efficiency of HIV prevention around the world: methods of the PANCEA project." *Health Services Research* 39 (6, part 2): 1993–2012.

Marseille, E., L. Dandona and others. 2007. "HIV prevention costs and program scale: data from the PANCEA project in five low and middle-income countries." *BMC Health Services Research* 7: 108.

Matovu, J. K., and others. 2002. "The Rakai Project counselling programme experience." *Tropical Medicine & International Health* 7 (12): 1064–1067.

Medlin, C., and D. de Walque. 2008. "Potential applications of conditional cash transfers for prevention of sexually transmitted infections and HIV in Sub-Saharan Africa." Policy Research Working Paper 4673. World Bank.

Menzies, N. A., and others. Forthcoming. "The cost of providing comprehensive HIV treatment in PEPFAR-supported programs." *AIDS*.

Miller, M. J., and others. 2000. "Sexual behavior changes and protease inhibitor therapy. SEROCO Study Group." *AIDS* 14 (4): F33–F39.

Montana, L. S., V. Mishra, and R. Hong. 2008. "Comparison of HIV Prevalence estimates from antenatal care surveillance and population-based surveys in sub-Saharan Africa." *British Medical Journal* 84 (Supplement 1): i78–i84.

Morris, M., and M. Kretzschmar. 1997. "Concurrent partnerships and the spread of HIV." *AIDS* 11 (5): 641–648.

Nachega, J. B., and others. 2010. "Association of antiretroviral therapy adherence and health care costs." *Annual Internal Medicine* 152 (1): 18–25.

National AIDS Control Council. 2007. *National HIV prevalence in Kenya* (Nairobi, July).

Oomman, N., D. Wendt, and C. Droggitis. 2010. *Zeroing In: AIDS Donors and Africa's Health Workforce*. HIV/AIDS Monitor Report. Center for Global Development.

Opio, A., and others. 2008. "Trends in HIV-related behaviors and knowledge in Uganda, 1989–2005: evidence of a shift toward more risk-taking behaviors." *Journal of Acquired Immune Deficiency Syndromes* 49 (3): 320–326.

Over, A. M. 1998. "The effects of societal variables on urban rates of HIV infection in developing countries." In *Confronting AIDS Evidence from the Developing World: Selected Background Papers for the World Bank Policy Research Report, Confronting AIDS: Public Priorities in a Global Epidemic*, edited by M. Ainsworth, L. Fransen, and A. M. Over. European Commission.

———. 2004. "Impact of the HIV/AIDS epidemic on the health sectors of developing countries." In *The Macroeconomics of HIV/AIDS*, edited by M. Haacker. International Monetary Fund.

———. 2008. "Prevention failure: the ballooning entitlement burden of U.S. global AIDS treatment spending and what to do about it." Working Paper 144. Center for Global Development.

————. 2009a. "AIDS treatment in South Asia: equity and efficiency arguments for shouldering the fiscal burden when prevalence rates are low." Working Paper 161. Center for Global Development.

————. 2009b. "Prevention failure: the ballooning entitlement burden of US Global AIDS treatment spending and what to do about it." *Revue d'Economie du Développement* 2009 (1–2): 107–144.

Over, A. M., and S. O. Aral. 2006. "The Economics of Sexually Transmitted Infections." *Sexually Transmitted Diseases* 33 (10): S79–S83.

Over, A. M., and P. Piot. 1996. "Human immunodeficiency virus infection and other sexually transmitted diseases in developing countries: public health importance and priorities for resource allocation." *Journal of Infectious Diseases* 174 (Supplement 2): S162–S175.

Over, A. M., and others. 2004. *HIV/AIDS Treatment and Prevention in India: Modeling the Costs and Consequences.* World Bank.

Over, A. M., E. Marseille, and others. 2006. "Antiretroviral therapy and HIV prevention in India: modeling costs and consequences of policy options." *Sexually Transmitted Diseases* 33 (10): S145–S152.

Over, A. M., A. Revenga and others. 2007. "The economics of effective AIDS treatment in Thailand." *AIDS* 21 (Supplement 4): S105–S116.

Packard, R. M. 1997. "Malaria dreams: postwar visions of health and development in the Third World." *Medical Anthropology* 17 (3): 279–296.

Padian, N. S., T. R. O'Brien, and others. 1993. "Prevention of heterosexual transmission of human immunodeficiency virus through couple counseling." *Journal of Acquired Immune Deficiency Syndrome* 6 (9): 1043–48.

Padian, N. S., and others. 2010. "Weighing the gold in the gold standard: challenges in HIV prevention research." *AIDS* 24 (5): 621–635.

Potts, M., and others. 2008. "Public health: reassessing HIV prevention." *Science* 320 (5877): 749–750.

Prescott, N. M. 1997. "Setting priorities for government involvement with antiretrovirals." In *Implications of Antiretroviral Treatment: Informal Consultation,* edited by E. van Praag, S. Fernyak, and A. M. Katz. World Health Organization.

Price, J., and others. 2007. "Integrating HIV clinical services in primary health centers in Rwanda: Effect on the quantity of non-HIV services delivered." PowerPoint presentation. Institute of Medicine. www.iom.edu/~/media/Files/ActivityFiles/Global/PEPFAR/PEPFARWSPPrice 5107.pdf.

Quinn, T. C., and others. 2000. "Viral load and heterosexual transmission of human immunodeficiency virus type 1." *New England Journal of Medicine* 342 (13): 921–929.

Radelet, Steven. 2003. *Challenging Foreign Aid: A Policymaker's Guide to the Millenium Challenge Account.* Center for Global Development.

Radelet, S., P. Abarcar, and R. Schutte. 2009. "What's behind the recent declines in U.S. foreign assistance?" Center for Global Development.

Ravishankar, N., and others. 2009. "Financing of global health: tracking development assistance for healthfrom 1990–2007." *The Lancet* 373 (9681): 2113–2124.

Revenga, A., and others. 2006. *The Economics of Effective AIDS Treatment: Evaluating Policy Options for Thailand.* World Bank.

Reynolds, H. W., M. J. Steiner, and W. Cates. 2005. "Contraception's proved potential to fight HIV." *Sexually Transmitted Infections* 81: 184–185.

Reynolds, H. W., and others. 2006. "The value of contraception to prevent perinatal HIV transmission." *Sexually Transmitted Diseases* 33 (6): 350–356.

Rosen, S., M. P. Fox, and C. J. Gill. 2007. "Patient retention in antiretroviral therapy programs in sub-Saharan Africa: a systematic review." *PLoS. Medicine* 4 (10): e298.

Roth, D. L., and others. 2001. "Sexual practices of HIV discordant and concordant couples in Rwanda: effects of a testing and counselling programme for men." *International Journal of STD &AIDS* 12 (3): 181–188.

Scitovsky, A. A., and A. M. Over. 1988. "AIDS: costs of care in the developed and the developing world." *AIDS* 2 (Supplement 1): S71–S81.

Sherr, L., and others. 2007. "Voluntary counselling and testing: uptake, impact on sexual behaviour, and HIV incidence in a rural Zimbabwean cohort." *AIDS* 21 (7): 851–860.

Soni, A., and R. Gupta. 2009. "Bridging the resource gap: improving value for money in HIV/AIDS treatment." *Health Affairs* 28 (6): 1617–1628.

Sorensen, J. L., and others. 2007. "Voucher reinforcement improves medication adherence in HIV-positive methadone patients: a randomized trial." *Drug and Alcohol Dependence* 88 (1): 54–63.

Stover, J., and others. 2003. "Adding family planning to PMTCT sites increases the benefits of PMTCT." Issue brief. U.S. Agency for International Development.

Sweat, M. D., and others. 2004. "Cost-effectiveness of nevirapine to prevent mother-to-child HIV transmission in eight African countries." *AIDS* 18 (12): 1661–1671.

Sweat, M. D., D. Kerrigan and others. 2006. "Cost-effectiveness of environmental-structural communication interventions for HIV prevention in the female sex industry in the Dominican Republic." *Journal of Health Communication* 11 (Supplement 2): 123–142.

Tanner, M., and D. de Savigny. 2008. "Malaria eradication back on the table." *Bulletin of the World Health Organization* 86 (2): 81–160.

Tarantola, D., and J. Mann. 1995. "AIDS and human rights." *AIDS and Society* 6 (4): 1, 5.

Tarantola, D., and others. 2006. "Jonathan Mann: founder of the health and human rights movement." *American Journal of Public Health* 96 (11): 1942–1943.

Thompson, W. 1929. "Population." *American Journal of Sociology* 34 (6): 959–975.

Thornton, Rebecca L. 2008. "The demand for, and impact of, learning HIV status." *American Economic Review* 98 (5): 1829–1863.

UNAIDS. 2007. *Financial Resources Required to Achieve Universal Access to HIV Prevention, Treatment, Care, and Support.*

———. 2008. *Report on the Global AIDS Epidemic, 2008.*

———. 2010. *Report on the Global AIDS Epidemic, 2010.*

Van Doorslaer, E., and others. 2006. "Effect of payments for health care on poverty estimates in 11 countries in Asia: an analysis of household survey data." *The Lancet* 368: 1357–1364.

Van Doorslaer, E., O. O'Donell and others. 2007. "Catastrophic payments for health care in Asia." *Health Economics* 16 (11): 1159–1184.

Van Doorslaer, E., A. Wagstaff, and F. F. H. Rutten. 1993. *Equity in the Finance and Delivery of Health Care: An International Perspective.* Oxford University Press.

van Praag, E., and J. H. Perriens. 1996. "Caring for patients with HIV and AIDS in middle income countries."*British Medical Journal* 313: 440.

Wagstaff, A. 2002. "Inequalities in health in developing countries: swimming against the tide?" Working Paper 2795. World Bank.

Wagstaff, A., E. Van Doorslaer, and P. Paci. 1989. "Equity in the finance and delivery of health care: some tentative cross-country comparisons." *Oxford Review of Economic Policy* 5 (1): 89–112.

Walker, D. G., M. Over, S. M. Bertozzi. Forthcoming. "Can studies of the cost of AIDS treatment improve the accountability of foreign assistance for health?" *AIDS.*

Wegbreit, J., and others. 2006. "Effectiveness of HIV prevention strategies in resource-poor countries: tailoring the intervention to the context." *AIDS* 20 (9): 1217–1235.

Weir, S. S., and others. 2002. "A pilot study of a rapid assessment method to identify places for AIDS prevention in Cape Town, South Africa." *Sexually Transmitted Infections* 78 (Supplement 1): i106–i113.

Weir, S. S., C. Pailman and others. 2003. "From people to places: focusing AIDS prevention efforts where it matters most." *AIDS* 17 (6): 895–903.

Weir, S. S., E. J. Tate, and others. 2004. "Where the action is: monitoring local trends in sexual behaviour." *Sexually Transmitted Infections* 80 (Supplement 2): ii63–ii68.

Were, W., and others. 2003. "Home-based model for HIV voluntary counselling and testing." *Lancet* 361 (9368): 1569.

Wester, C. W., and others. 2009. "Adult combination antiretroviral therapy in sub-Saharan Africa: lessons from Botswana and future challenges." *HIV Therapy* 3 (5): 501–526.

When to Start Consortium and Jonathan Sterne. 2009. "Timing of initiation of antiretroviral therapy in AIDS-free HIV-1-infected patients: a collaborative analysis of 18 HIV cohort studies." *Lancet* 373 (9672): 1352–1363.

White, P. 2007. *Improving Parameter Estimation, Projection Methods, Uncertainty Estimation, and Epidemic Classification: Report of a Meeting of the UNAIDS Reference Group on Estimates, Modelling and Projections held in Prague, Czech Republic, November 29th–December 1st 2006*. Geneva, Switzerland: UNAIDS.

Wilson, D., and D. T. Halperin. 2008. "'Know your epidemic, know your response': a useful approach, if we get it right." *Lancet* 372 (9637): 423–426.

World Bank. 1993. *Investing in Health*.

WHO (World Health Organization). 2006. *Antiretroviral Therapy for HIV Infection in Adults and Adolescents*. HIV/AIDS Program.

———. 2009. *Rapid Advice: Antiretroviral Therapy for HIV Infection in Adults and Adolescents*.

WHO, UNAIDS, and UNICEF. 2007. *Towards Universal Access: Scaling Up Priority HIV/AIDS Interventions in the Health Sector. Progress Report 2007*. www.who.int/hiv/mediacentre/universal_access_progress_report_en. pdf.

———. 2009. *Towards Universal Access: Scaling Up Priority HIV/AIDS Interventions in the Health Sector. Progress Report 2009*. www.who.int/hiv/pub/2009progressreport/en/.

———. 2010. *Towards Universal Access: Scaling Up Priority HIV/AIDS Interventions in the Health Sector. Progress Report 2010*. www.who.int/hiv/pub/2010progressreport/report/en/index.html.

Index

The Center for Global Development

The Center for Global Development works to reduce global poverty and inequality through rigorous research and active engagement with the policy community to make the world a more prosperous, just, and safe place for us all. The policies and practices of the rich and the powerful—in rich nations, as well as in the emerging powers, international institutions, and global corporations—have significant impacts on the world's poor people. We aim to improve these policies and practices through research and policy engagement to expand opportunities, reduce inequalities, and improve lives everywhere. By pairing research with action, CGD goes beyond contributing to knowledge about development. We conceive of and advocate for practical policy innovations in areas such as trade, aid, health, education, climate change, labor mobility, private investment, access to finance, and global governance to foster shared prosperity in an increasingly interdependent world.